Doctor Schiff's
Miracle Weight-Loss Guide

Martin M. Schiff, M.D.

Doctor Schiff's
Miracle Weight-Loss Guide

Parker Publishing Company, Inc. **West Nyack, N.Y.**

Library of Congress Cataloging in Publication Data

Schiff, Martin M
    Doctor Schiff's miracle weight-loss guide.

    1. Reducing diets. I. Title. II. Title:
Miracle weight-loss guide. [DNLM: 1. Diet, Reducing.
2. Obesity--Therapy--Popular works. WD212 S331d]
Rm222.2.S268   613.2'5   74-13147
ISBN 0-13-217026-4

Dedication

To my wife, Millie, for her help, love and understanding. To dream the dream, strengthened by our children, Michael, David, Denise, and Howard. To Grandma Celia and Grandpa Irving Tepley who are the rocks of our Gibraltar.

HOW THIS BOOK WILL HELP
YOU CONTROL YOUR WEIGHT

True or false?—"Food has made me fat. Cutting down on food will make me thin."

False. If it were true, you would not be reading this page. The fact that diets are an illusion is now dawning on millions of rotund dieters who lose (and regain) scores of pounds each year.

Cutting down on food is like taking an aspirin for chronic pain. It is a temporary measure.

My patients lose weight and fat permanently. And they never miss a meal. True or false?—"I have made myself fat. I can make myself thin."

True.

You should be glad to hear this, but many of you won't exactly be jumping with joy. We often place the blame for our misery on anybody or anything except ourselves.

But there's a good side to it. You hold the reins. You can decide whether you will continue on the groaning see-saw of lose and gain or alight on the solid ground of youthful, good looks once and for all.

If you choose the latter, this is your book. I'll tell you why I think so.

I'm not a psychiatrist. I'm not a psychologist. I am a family-type physician. I might even say "old-fashioned" family-type physician. But I won't. Still, I'm tempted because I want you to understand that I have an interest in you personally. With me there's no fast shuffle. The more you weigh, the more interest I have in you.

That's why I specialize in bariatrics—helping overweight people.

I used to prescribe diets. I don't anymore. I have something much better. All you have to be willing to do is learn to know yourself. Eating is only a small part of it. Thinking is a major part of it.

Thinking about what? Thinking about you, about your potential for being admired, being influential, being capable, being physically irresistible. Thinking about what you're thinking about. Reprograming yourself by a simple two-step method. Changing negative thoughts, feelings and emotions into those that are positive, creative of your goals, and success-oriented.

Applied to that tenacious, stubborn disease known as obesity, or even to those mere ten or twenty pounds of excess baggage, the results are exquisitely satisfying.

Lose from 1 to 7 pounds a week without willpower or hunger . . . Never count another calorie . . . Enjoy normal, healthful dining . . . Eat six times a day and more, if you wish . . . Never go on a diet again.

If you would first like to fill your belly with a lusty steak smothered in mushrooms or a roast chicken dinner, go ahead.

It's part of the program.

Why do I call this a "miracle" guide? Because everyone who reads and utilizes this book is capable of developing and producing a miracle within themselves.

I don't perform a miracle. It is you yourself, programing and reprograming day by day, who makes a miracle. You do this through your own well-directed efforts, purposeful determination and hard work—that is actually a labor of love.

Eventually you will find this work easier and easier. You will become more at ease with yourself and develop *perfect* weight control. Eventually *you* will be the MIRACLE!

Thousands have found this a fascinating adventure as they watched themselves grow thin before their very eyes.

It is self-awareness, self programing, self-understanding, self-discovery, all rolled into one exciting, dynamic success story.

It is learning to be your own best friend and to love yourself.

It is a physical change (pounds and inches).

It is a mental, psychological, emotional, spiritual transformation—a MIRACLE!

Martin M. Schiff, M.D.

Acknowledgement

To my office staff—Bertha, Linda, Carol and Kathy, a special thanks for their encouragement, support and ever helpful suggestions. To my many patients whose miracles allow the sun to penetrate the covers of this book. Thus, a warmer, clearer, brighter picture of what IT is all about.

CONTENTS

6. PITFALLS INTO WHICH FAT PEOPLE FALL THE
HARDEST *(Continued)*

7. HOW TO DEVELOP A MENTAL "SET" THAT PROGRAMS YOU
FOR SLENDERIZING SUCCESS 120

8. END FAULTY EATING HABITS, BEGIN SLENDERIZING
HABITS PRACTICALLY INSTANTLY WITH SELF-HYPNOSIS 135

11. TEN STEPS TO A GREAT NEW SLENDER LIFE *(Continued)*

12. HOW TO MAINTAIN YOUR BODY AT ITS ATTRACTIVE BEST WITHOUT A SECOND THOUGHT 200

Doctor Schiff's
Miracle Weight-Loss Guide

1

THE HIDDEN REASON WHY YOU ARE
NOT AS SLIM AS YOU WOULD LIKE TO BE

This is a diet book.

But you would never know it.

A better description is: A no-diet, weight-loss program.

It shows you how to eat well and not to be concerned about how much or how fast you are losing weight.

Yet, thousands of my patients who have been on my program have shed as much as thirty to forty pounds in a month . . . without half trying.

The psychologists have a concept they call the law of diminishing effect: The harder you try the more likely you are to fail.

This is so true—especially when it comes to dieting to lose weight. There is no "trying" in my program. Therefore, it is not a trying program. Instead, it is fun.

If it is fun to lose weight—more fun than it is to gain weight—how can you miss? If you can lose weight even with a full belly, isn't your success assured?

THE MIRACLE KEY TO PERMANENT WEIGHT LOSS

The key is in you. However. . .

I can't tell you very much about that key at this time as it is different for everyone. But. . .

This book can tell you how to find this key, how to place it in the keyhole of your excess weight and how to open the door to a new, slender, attractive body—yours to enjoy for the duration of a longer, happier life.

I have helped thousands of overweight people to do this. They are now beautiful people. They range from models and steward-esses anxious to drop those ten stubborn pounds, to mothers with a hundred pounds of unwanted fat burdening their steps; from Hollywood actors with a slight paunch to flatten out, to executives with an 80-inch corporation.

They reached their weight goal, and they stay slim. I seldom have to see them again regarding their weight problems.

Once you find the key to your slender self, the weight problem that has plagued you all these years is no longer a problem.

AN INSIDE LOOK AT MY PROFESSIONAL PRACTICE

Were you to visit my Los Angeles office, you would see me in quiet, personal conversations with my patients. I don't allow a desk to come between us. We sit knee to knee and eyeball to eyeball. We are friends.

Want to eavesdrop?

Her husband was OK until . . .

"My husband is an easy-going type. He is happy with just a roof over his head. I'm a girl used to the nice things in life. We are happy, but my pregnancy went wrong and after the surgery I gained 60 pounds. Now my weight is beginning to affect my marriage. We adopted a girl seven months ago. But my weight is still going up. Now my husband says I must lose weight—or else!"

You see me taking notes. I need these notes to help her find the key. I explain she must come to a three-hour orientation lecture, all the important aspects of which are presented in this book. Most of my new patients attend this lecture.

I move to another consultation room.

She loved sweets so much

"I eat all day long, not what's good for me but sweets such as candy and cake. My mother has the same trouble. I'm not the only one."

"But you are the one with the weight problem and coming to me for help."

"Right, so what do I do? I love sweets so."

"But do you love yourself?"

"Doc, you know, I'm killing myself slowly. Maybe I don't. Yet, I'm proud of everything I do."

"Are you proud of your eating and your weight?"

"No, I don't want to be fat."

A successful salesman's situation

Look and listen through another keyhole.

A salesman is explaining, "For the past two years I've been sitting behind the wheel of my Mark IV or behind a luxurious luncheon spread, talking with my customers. I live off the fat of the land."

Some miscellaneous cases

Then, in another consultation room, a 29-year old single woman who is a student at UCLA is in tears as she tells me, "I don't think I'm accomplishing anything. One lousy pound all week. I want to do things and move on to something better."

I stay cool. "Patience. Allow yourself time."

You hear a woman say, "When my mother died, I blamed myself. I had guilt feelings and punished myself. Now I'm tired of being fat. I want to lose weight and feel better."

And another, "I think it's time for me to stop making food a purpose or a substitute."

Is this all just a lot of talk?

Maybe.

But *it's people thinking and talking themselves thin.*

WHY MY SYSTEM BEATS "DIETING"

When you think about overeating, and fight it, you eventually surrender.

The harder you try by dieting, by willpower, by aimless determination, the surer you are to lose and gain, lose and gain.

You just perpetuate the problem.

I'm not saying you shouldn't eat properly. I help you to eat in a balanced, nonfattening way in this book.

But what is far more important, I help you to discover yourself.

When you learn to know yourself, you understand yourself. When you understand yourself, the problem within you stops screaming for understanding.

Usually, a problem's scream is drowned in the squeaking of a refrigerator door or the tinkle of glasses.

No problem—no overweight.

If you look at dieting with a clear viewpoint, temporary starvation is really a farce. You gain nothing, except your weight back—eventually.

It's treating the symptom, not the cause.

It is fun to treat the cause. It's similar to an inner adventure—a mental safari.

And the rewards are immense. You become the guy or girl you have always admired who doesn't have an overweight problem.

Did you ever stop to realize when you diet that you need other people's cooperation? It's not a solo trip such as you may think. But do they cooperate? Forget it. They work against you. Hard.

"Aw, c'mon. One slice won't hurt you. Baked it myself."

When you diet, you receive no sympathy from family or friends. Here, as never before, you need encouragement. But what actually happens? You receive invitations to cocktail parties, barbeques and dinner parties. Jokes about the look on your face when they eat or drink in front of you and miscellaneous mirth about your girth.

Even strangers sense you're on a diet. You are offered candy by children, cookies by someone in the elevator. The people at the next table in the restaurant seem to flaunt their French pastry at you.

Diets require the cooperation of other people. That's why groups such as Weight Watchers and Take Off Pounds Sensibly (TOPS) have more success than individuals on their own.

But learning to know yourself is a private affair. Other people cannot try, tempt or taunt you. No one else knows you're on a weight loss program. You don't need their cooperation.

It's between you and you, I and Me.

You lift the veil between you and your inner self.

Somewhere there is a mental "weight" causing physical weight.

You have a group of two: Your conscious and subconscious mind.

A good name for your "group" might be Weight Lifters!

"Doctor, I can see results. I was down in the dumps when I began. I find it easier each day to think and learn about 'me.' I am losing inches. Clothes fit looser. People are noticing. I like myself better. I feel great."

I have heard that a thousand times.

Often benefits far exceed pounds lost. A.J., 29, had gained weight since her divorce. When she started the program she weighed 131. In six weeks she weighed 112. This was the least of the benefits.

- She had been dating a much younger man and there were emotional problems. She broke off with him and was much happier dating others.
- She returned to the teaching profession after a two-year absence.
- She let her hair go natural and dressed more tastefully.
- Her drawn, unhappy face became more relaxed, smiling, youthful looking.
- She stopped smoking pot.
- She became less withdrawn, more talkative and outgoing.

Often pounds gained are part of a broader syndrome. Attack only the pounds, leaving the cause of the syndrome intact, and you may miss the experience of a great new life. You also could gain the pounds back.

What a difference a few pounds can make in your love life. I'll never forget the transformation in J.S., 36, a divorcee. She came in the first day sloppily dressed, her teeth in as poor shape as the rest of her body.

In two months, weighing 120 instead of 151, J.S. had extensive dental work done. Then she had her long stringy hair cut feather-style. Then she began wearing cute clothes—short skirts, hot pants, boots. She started bowling, skin diving, met a guy and eventually married him.

Flo Ziegfeld, producer of the famous Follies of a half-century ago, had a sign on his stage door—"Through these portals pass the most beautiful girls in the world." I may do the same on my office door some day. Only I would add the words . . . "on the way out."

The actuarial tables show you live longer if you weigh less. I don't have to consult these tables to know the health benefits derived from a few pounds off.

I see patients with arthritis straighten up.

I see blood pressure drop and candidates for heart trouble lose their hypertension.

I see skin, hair, and nails brighten.

I see all sorts of leg complaints and back problems disappear.

I see the end of colitis, intestinal problems, ulcers, etc.

I see blood sugar in diabetics drop. Example: A woman, 50, who lost 28 pounds in five months saw her blood sugar level drop from 393 MG/100ML to 187. Her insulin dosage was reduced and, of course, the blood sugar level increased temporarily; then dropped to 152—a great morale booster for her.

HOW YOUR MENTAL CHEMISTRY CONTROLS
YOUR BODY CHEMISTRY

If you *knew* what a magnificent person you were—how you have the ability to make as much money as you want, as many friends, attract love, invent, create—you would not be reading this book.

You would be healthy, slim, youthful in appearance. We all become the person we know or see ourselves to be.

You are the person you *know* yourself to be.

Who is really brainwashing you?

"Stupid! You've broken another glass."

We are brainwashed to think less of ourselves. The brainwashers are usually our parents, our teachers, our friends and our co-workers. But the biggest brainwasher is you.

You create an image of yourself in your own mind as unattractive, or unable, or un-something. And so you become.

Once you are overweight, you tend to develop an overweight image of yourself which helps to keep you overweight. But seldom does overweight begin that way. Usually, you have a limited or negative self-image in some other way. This detracts from your satisfaction or pleasure in life, so you substitute by seeking extra oral pleasure. The excess poundage had derived from your negative self-image, indirectly.

Remember that famous cartoon? The psychiatrist is telling the patient, "The reason you have an inferiority complex is that you *are* inferior."

Witty but inaccurate. A person with shortcomings is more likely to compensate for them by being a braggard. The point is that we do behave according to our self-image.

Even your body follows your mind. Worry produces ulcers. Fear makes the heart beat faster and the sweat glands overactive. Anxiety causes tension which in turn produces dis-ease.

Emotions and attitudes affect our appetite for food. They also control our true hunger by affecting our metabolism. But it's appetite, more often than hunger, that drives us to the candy box or cookie jar.

One middle-aged man did not enjoy the work he was doing. He gained steadily during this period becoming portly and ungainly in appearance. Then he had the opportunity to go into a business he enjoyed. He began to lose weight. Within six months he had lost fifty pounds. "Nothing changed about my eating," he explained later. "I just lost my taste for ice cream." He had been eating one or two quarts of the stuff a day. Apparently, an "appetite" for tasty ice cream arose from his tasteless work.

IT ISN'T ONLY FOOD THAT MAKES YOU FAT

On the pages ahead we will explore how matters totally unrelated to food are behind overweight problems. We will see how the simple act of identifying these matters often eliminates their effects on us—and pounds disappear from our arms, waist, thighs, etc.

"But I have no problems, Doc." I hear this often.

"OK, you have no problems. But do you admit your body has a problem?"

"Sure, or I wouldn't be here."

"Then what causes your body's overweight problem?"

"Glands, maybe?"

"And, if this is so, what causes your glands to give you problems?"

"I guess it's heredity."

What this person is saying is "It's not my fault. It's not my fault. It's not my fault."

Well, I have bad news for the overweight egotist who is not to blame for being fat: It *is* your fault.

Organic disorders are the cause of obesity less than 1 percent of the time. Rather, obesity is often the cause of the organic disorders.

It may be painful for some people to realize it is their fault they are overweight. But look at it as good news. If you are the cause, then you can also be the cure.

To those who say, "I have no problems, Doctor," I say, "OK, you have no problems. But watch those pounds disappear as you move ahead on this miracle weight-loss program."

CHANGING YOUR MENTAL CHEMISTRY PAYS OFF IN POUNDS OFF

Often we are not aware we are being "bugged" by our mental attitudes. Something we experienced years ago, and long since forgotten—at least consciously—is still residing in our subconscious mind and pulling physiological strings—often to our detriment.

We are the puppets of our own past programing—until we learn to pull the strings ourselves.

There is no one way to learn this. I provide you with many methods. Often, the very act of paying attention to ourselves will solve the problem. False appetites disappear and we begin to lose weight. Sometimes we reverse the weight trend without actually knowing why, any more than we knew why when we began to overeat.

How do you pay attention to yourself?

Following is the case of one young woman, 22, and overweight, keeping a diary:

"Wednesday I did not go to class. I bought a newspaper and remained in my room. Three locks on my door—all of them locked. I lifted the phone off the hook and placed the receiver in a drawer. Even though the moon was in Leo. The paper said a girl had been raped and stabbed the night before off a main highway. Her body had been found down a canyon a little distance from her car. I lit a candle and didn't go outside. Not even to the grocery store. My phone whined insistently from within the drawer.

"Oysters make a nice midnight or early morning snack. They have fewer calories than clams but are more expensive—probably because they contain pearls. . . . In the mornings I cannot always recall whether I actually ate them or if it was a dream. Not until I notice the empty can sitting around somewhere, the spoon still in it. Vague memories of crunching on an occasional grain of sand. Or as often as not, I wake up next to a cold, damp, apple core.

"Monday the moon is in Scorpio and I miss my morning class again. Dark, mysterious Scorpio, ruled by Mars, god of vengeance. I dress in a heavy coat to drive to my night class. It ends at quarter of ten. The twenty-minute drive home is along a dark highway. My car is steering oddly. I pull off to check the problem. Hissing in my right front tire. Someone has punctured it with a screw. Someone wants to kill me. A van pulls up and a man climbs out. I cannot see his face. I jump in the car—lock the doors. His headlights light up his face as he turns back to his van. I stay in the car until morning. When the moon comes into Sagittarius."

Can you feel her fear and insecurity? Can you see a connection with her excess weight?

Do you think this person was gaining insight about herself by writing? When she read this over later, she recalls, she wondered if the tire was actually flat. The subconscious mind can operate our behavior in many ways.

You don't have to write to pay attention to yourself. But writing is one way and for some an enjoyable way. I encourage my patients to write, especially letters. "I'm writing a book," I explain. "Perhaps your letter will be in the book." And they write reams. As the ink supply decreases, so does their weight.

One obese patient's writing experience

Here is a letter from one 32-year old woman who did not see the point in writing. She weighed 199 when she first saw me in September. By the following February she had lost only 18 pounds.

Then she began to write.

"I sat here for a long time with a blank piece of paper in the typewriter. I've gained weight. I'm ashamed. I want to run away and hide but I can't. I can't stand to carry this weight around so I must come back. I must listen. I must learn and I must change my habits. If I don't, when I finally shed the weight I wish to lose, it will return again.

"In a rating of from 0 to 100 I would rate myself less than 0. I hate fat people. I'm fat. I hate myself. When I see a fat person I think 'how disgusting' . . . I suppose people think that when they see me too. I'm afraid to leave the apartment in fear someone will think this, yet I know you've said I care too much about what other people think. In reality I know people could care less one way or another about me . . . but it doesn't make the feeling go away.

"My husband is an alcoholic. I don't like the word any more than I like the word fat but it is true in both cases. Many people ask, 'Why do you stay with an alcoholic?' I think, 'Why does he stay with me?' Our problems are so similar. We (eat/drink) indulge for the same reasons or at least similar ones.

"As I grew older I guess I began to accept his going out once a week (sometimes twice a week) and coming home a mess—smelling horrible and his hands shaking, shaking, shaking. I'm so afraid of his destroying himself.

"In everything I write to you over and over again you can see this same pattern of thinking . . . always worried about what the other person thinks about me, my husband, my marriage, my children. Now I'm going to listen to what I think. . ."

She did listen (to herself). She did learn. And she finally began to lose those bulges when she got to know herself better.

Writing can pay off in pounds off.

INSIDE EVERY OVERWEIGHT PERSON IS A SLIM PERSON TRYING TO CLIMB OUT

When you begin to gain insight about yourself—whether it is by thinking, writing, or other methods we will go into—you begin to see that your true self is a slender person.

You wonder how this slender person became mired in all that fat.

You begin to free yourself of those chubby chains.

That's the breakthrough.

Once you see yourself, not as others see you, but as the inner person you actually are, you begin to become that person externally.

What it boils down to is: see yourself the slender person you actually are and the fat on you melts away.

Believe my thousands of slender ex-patients: It beats dieting.

How does my system work?

Once you begin to *be* the inner person who is the real you masquerading as a fat person, your behavior patterns change.

Behavior modification techniques are now being looked upon with more and more favor by many physicians. Eating at certain times, in certain places, and in certain ways helps you to *be* the inner person by abandoning the old behavior patterns of the fake, fat self.

One physician I know prescribes appetite suppression tablets to help his obese patients decrease their intake. He then watches the progress. If the weight loss ceases, he discontinues the pills, explaining "Obviously, the pills are not working." This is like punishment. Rewards and punishment are used in this way to modify behavior.

You and I will be a little more subtle in the use of rewards and punishment, if we use them at all. What we are more interested in doing to modify behavior is to minimize our exposure to old, negative habits and conditionings and replace them with new, positive habits and behavior patterns which fit the slender life style.

I have an easy, fun way for you to do this. You'll enjoy letting go and watching it happen.

You will find yourself walking past the refrigerator and never seeing it.

"You cannot work into this program just by thinking about it," said one young man. "When I arrive home from work, I'm in the habit of eating. If I only thought about it, it wouldn't be five minutes and I'd be in the refrigerator. So I sit down and write. Writing helps with the transition of work to home. Gradually, my craving for food passes. Then when I do eat, I'm satisfied with less. Reading or hearing about others doing this isn't enough. You have to do it to appreciate it."

Weight loss can be rapid. A.S. weighed 274 which he carried quite well on his 6'4" frame. But, as a business manager for a hospital, he was reminded time and time again about his excess baggage. Here is his record:

Date	Weight	
4/22/71	274	
5/13/71	253	(21 pounds off in 3 weeks)
5/27/71	242	(11 pounds off in 2 weeks)
6/10/71	228	(14 pounds off in 2 weeks)
6/24/71	215	(13 pounds off in 2 weeks)
7/8/71	206	(9 pounds off in 2 weeks)
8/19/71	191	(15 pounds off in 6 weeks)

In 11 weeks he dropped 68 pounds. In 17 weeks he shed 83 pounds!

On this program your measurements seem to change where change is needed. A fat behind is first to go. Or, if a woman's abdomen is the storage area, the largest measurement changes will usually occur there. K.R. was a 5'7" housewife who was heavy all over. Here is how her measurements changed over a three-month period as she went from 186 to 143 pounds:

	Bust	Waist	Hips	Thighs
	42	36	44	25
	38	29½	37	20
Inches lost	4"	6½"	7"	5"

The body seems to know what is normal and pares down in the desired places.

HOW TO CREATE YOUR OWN THINK TANK
FOR WEIGHT REDUCTION

The Rand Corporation in Santa Monica, California, was created by Douglas Aircraft in 1946 to begin "a program of study and research on the broad subject of intercontinental warfare." Today there are 15,000 of these "think tanks" devoted to research and development in many areas.

The most popular of these areas is the human being. Entire societies are examined as well as the behavior of individuals. At Stanford Research Institute, near San Francisco, monkeys are outfitted with artificial brains to learn more about how the mind works.

Each one of us is a think tank, actually. Even when our conscious mind is asleep, another think tank that never sleeps is still operating: the subconscious mind, like a computer, runs our body, activating certain glands and secretions at the precise time, keeping our lungs moving and our heart beating.

This automatic part of our mind can work at cross purposes with our conscious think tank. Or, the two can be "pals."

The person who consciously wants to quit smoking but who is impelled to light up by habit finds his two think tanks working against each other.

There are ways to make your conscious and subconscious minds become pals. I'll show you how later.

Once you align your conscious and subconscious minds, things go great for you. You have peace of mind. Your health improves. Your eating patterns become normal.

And your weight returns to normal.

THE MEANING OF MIND-BODY IN LOSING WEIGHT

A young lady came to my office. She was 22 years old, 5'2", and weighed 142 pounds. She said she was setting her goal at 118 pounds. 1 recorded her basic "history," gave her recipes, etc. and started her on the program.

She seemed delighted at the idea of writing. When she returned she brought me the following. 1 want you to read it now and play psychiatrist for this girl. Some phrases are real giveaways. Can you spot them?

"When I was much younger, I had to wear glasses because my eyes crossed. My older brother never wanted me around. Maybe he was disappointed I was a girl instead of a boy.

"Michele was born two years after me. My mother tells me I was very jealous. I dropped books and teddy bears on her; tried to throw her in the trash can. I started wetting my bed soon after she was born, perhaps in rebellion. John came along two years later—Philip three years after that.

"I was always extremely sensitive and easily hurt. My father could make me burst into tears by simply looking at me. Older brother, Sam, discovered this immediately and capitalized on it.

"I was always accused of gorging at meals and in between, the chubby one that no one liked. So I began feeling guilty about eating. I really wanted Sam to like me but I believed what he said. I was the outcast of the family, the chubby one who wet her bed, wore glasses and ate too much.

"Also, I had many problems with my health and teeth. It is possible that my health problems were a bid for attention and teeth problems a result of Father's ominous forecast I would 'grow up to be a toothless old hag' if I didn't brush my teeth.

"My mother was a beautiful model. People would ask what happened to me. I can still feel the resentment. Why did I have to be the ugly duckling in such a beautiful family? Mom teased me when I started developing and I withdrew. I took refuge in food. Wore my trainer bra to bed at night hoping it would keep me a little girl. Refused to accept the fact that I was becoming a woman.

"I used to eat my lunch in the bathroom at school in the 7th grade—in one of the stalls. Convinced myself that I didn't need anyone. I was above them. But I wanted them to like me. Tried to be something I wasn't—makeup, hair style, stockings at school. At home, just myself alone, with food.

"I quit wetting my bed at twelve but sometime back developed the habit of midnight snacking. When nobody was watching, I would cram my mouth with giant bites of food. Ice cream, cookies, milk, anything and everything. Sometimes I would go back to bed and forget about it completely the next day. I'd find the evidence in bed with me—a banana skin, cookie crumbs, one time a half eaten box of cake mix.

"My mother warned me I was turning my body into a garbage can. It was almost a ritual, sort of trance-like. No memory of it the next day."

This patient wrote more in subsequent days; however, the account of her early years is especially revealing. I'm sure you noted the following facts as possible clues as to why her present emotional profile is giving her a fat profile.

Analysis of above case

- She felt her older brother wanted her to be a boy.
- She was jealous of the attention given her younger sister and brothers.
- She refused to accept the fact that she was becoming a woman.
- She didn't need anyone and found companionship in food.

You could probably add to this list.

Remember, although this is about her youth some ten to fifteen years ago, it is written today. So it reflects her feelings today to the extent these feelings have been carried over from yesterday.

I could see she was still that 12-year old girl in many ways. I encouraged her to think and write. The more she thought, the more she wrote, and the more she wrote, the less she weighed.

She literally wrote her weight off!

Your mind controls your body.

Your mind makes you overweight.

Your mind can make you thin.

THE PART FOOD PLAYS IN YOUR WEIGHT PROBLEM

Don't misunderstand me.

Food plays an important part in your weight problem.

Your mind can bring you to alcohol or to kleptomania or to becoming a golf-aholic.

However, it has brought *you* to food. You may be overeating because you are under-somethingelsing. Still, food is very much involved. In a way, food is a symptom and not the cause.

So we treat the symptom almost as you would treat the pain of a headache. You take the aspirin and kill the pain first. Then you reason why you were tense and what you can do about it.

The first thing to do

The very first thing I will do is help you select foods that nourish more than they fatten you.

The odds are you seek oral gratification rather than hunger gratification when you eat. You lean instinctively toward the crisp, the crunchy and the sweet.

To me crisp, crunchy and sweet food spells fats and carbohydrates.

Now wouldn't it be a great world for such eaters if fats, starches and sugars built bones, muscles and vital organs.

The fact of life is—they build fat.

Proteins are the nutrients that build the body's structure and keep it vital and renewed. We also derive energy from protein.

Proteins are meats, poultry, fish, eggs.

The huge sprawling carbohydrate industry—the bakers, pizza parlors and candy makers would have us believe they are in an essential business: providing our body with energy-giving foods.

True, they give us energy, but not very much of essential body nourishment.

On the other hand, foods that give our body nourishment also give energy. *Proteins can be complete foods. Sweets and starches can never be complete foods.*

I'm not going to ask you to count calories.

I'm not going to ask you to skip meals.

I'm not going to ask you to diet.

I'm not going to ask you to go hungry for one single minute.

I *am* going to ask you to adjust food intake in order to gradually reach your weight goal.

I *am* going to ask you to trade me your breakfast pastry for a couple of eggs, any style. Your luncheon hamburger for a hamburger steak. Your dinner spaghetti for broiled fish. Your leftover pie snack for a cold chicken leg.

I *am* going to ask you to switch from sweets and starches to lusty proteins—*to stop feeding your mouth and start feeding your body.*

Here's the Big Switch:

AWAY FROM	TO
Doughnuts	Hamburger steak
Pastry	Lamb
Cereals	All cuts of beef
Crackers	Veal
Bread and rolls	Fish
Cake	Seafood (clams, etc.)
Spaghetti	Chicken
Pizza, pasta	Turkey (and other poultry)
Ice cream	Eggs
Pie	Cheeses
Candy	Low calorie drinks
Sweet drinks	Salads and leafy vegetables

This is all I ask of you in the area of that dirty word—*diet.* I limit the use of that word in this book. It is misleading.

You don't diet. You switch some foods. But you don't deprive yourself or fall into that carrot stick-celery-melba toast syndrome.

In fact, you will never use the word "diet" again if you follow the program in this book.

YOUR BURNING DESIRE TO BE THIN CAN MELT FAT AWAY

My program cannot help you if you are happy to be the way you are. You must want to change.

Your desire to change means that every now and then you will set this book aside and do some of the things prescribed.

Such as think.

That's the main activity called for. But I promise you it won't be thinking, such as Calculus or Philosophy or the History of Religion. Maybe close to Psychology.

It is not heavy thinking. It is fun thinking because it's about you.

There are other things to do. For example, relax and see (visualize) certain pictures in your mind. This affects your behavior. No aimless discipline, no willpower. Just sitting comfortably and imagining. It is called mental reprograming. Visualize yourself slender, then you unconsciously change your behavior and become the person you see.

So you become a think tank oriented to yourself and able to carry out effortlessly the changes proposed by your think tank.

If the food switches described a page ago appear difficult at first glance today, they can become the most natural thing in the world tomorrow. Through reprograming.

A patient said to me, "I'm not too anxious to look inside me. I'm afraid of what I may find."

The story of Pandora's Box, symbolic of the memories stored in the mind, is not a happy one. But I promised this man, as I promise you, there are many positive thoughts and ideas of which you can be proud, stored in your mind, other than the negative hang-ups.

You may have to step on one or two ugly events in your life. But you will step up scores of strong points about yourself, abilities and talents—all sources of immense satisfaction which are presently being suppressed.

On the pages ahead you will open a Pandora's Box full of priceless treasures—all yours.

You will find you are a most attractive person. Also, there is no one exactly like you in the entire world.

In the Box will be gifts of talent, of gab, and of versatility. You will acquire new energy, new popularity, new wisdom.

With these gifts you will begin a new life of fun, success, health, and meaning.

You stand on the threshold of that new life at this very moment.

The Meat of Chapter 1

So you thought food was your basic problem.

No way.

Food is merely one of your body's reactions to your basic problem.

You may be unable to solve the problem but you can eliminate the food reaction.

The food reaction makes you overweight and leads to more problems.

If you pay attention to yourself, you begin to identify the basic problem. Then you can change the eating reaction to it.

Pay attention by thinking and writing about your thoughts. Be your own think tank.

Meanwhile, make the Big Switch. Don't cut down. Substitute.

My name is Dr. Schiff. What's yours? Now let's look beneath the name in order to know and understand each other.

2

HOW TO LOSE 10, 25, 50 POUNDS
OF UNWANTED BULGE EFFORTLESSLY

Appetizer for Chapter 2

Words can be fattening.

You are reading me correctly. The words you speak can help make you overweight.

The language you use can program you for weight loss or weight gain.

There are problem words which perpetuate problems and may even create new problems.

There are solution words which end problems and produce new, more acceptable conditions.

Solution words lead to changed attitudes. In this chapter you learn the power of the mind over calories, how to derive more pleasure from the food you eat, and what actually rings your appetite bell.

Watch for 25 tips—so the pew won't tip when you sit down in church.

If you can derive more fun out of life, you won't need as much fun from food.

This is a fun book. You and I are going to have a "helluvva" good time.

35

Calorie counters are fun spoilers. Calories count, but you won't count them. Forget calorie-counting.

Scales are killjoys. You won't have to remind yourself how little you have lost by hopping on a scale every few hours. Forget scales, except maybe once or twice a week.

Small portions are for the birds. No snacking between meals is for prisoners. Special menues are for sick people. Forget them all.

You will have fun eating without regrets.

But you won't depend on eating for your fun.

Mis-directed, repetitious effort is the biggest bore of all. Exerting aimless effort or willpower as a way of life is doomed to failure and to self-recrimination. You and I don't accept failure and we don't berate ourselves.

We do believe in the positive approach—positive thinking, and positive actions.

The reason we are so positive about this is: Negativity is depressing—it tends to depress or lower one's metabolism and as one burns fewer calories, one stores more fat.

On the other hand, positivity is elevating. It tends to raise enthusiasm and metabolism. One burns more calories, stores less fat.

HOW THE WORDS YOU USE CAN AFFECT YOUR WEIGHT

"I've tried all kinds of diets but they just don't work."

This man was trying to sell me a bill of goods but I wasn't buying.

"You are setting yourself up for another failure, as you now have to prove this statement is correct."

"But, Doc, I'm discouraged."

He was discouraged alright. About his becoming a father coupled with a recent layoff from his job. And he was taking it out on food. I gave him a special project.

"When you come back in two weeks, bring me a list of all the encouraging aspects in your life. Each time you think the list is complete, add another item to it."

He did his homework well. The list was a long one. He had a twinkle in his eye when he handed it to me. I showed him how to use the list in programing himself for optimism and expectation, especially in becoming his true slender self. I was so optimistic myself, I neglected to weigh him that day.

Words are a tip off as to "where your head is at."

"My eating is out of control. I go on binges."

Can eating ever be out of control? What this person is actually saying is, "Eating is top priority to me at this point in my life." Under this condition it is easier to shuffle priorities rather than control eating.

"When I watch TV, I often feel a sudden craving to eat something I shouldn't."

Is this person associating TV with the illicit? Probing may reveal that TV had been allowed in earlier years only when homework was completed. But, when the folks were not around to check .... Possible mental "reset": I can watch TV or eat any time I want. Before I do, though, I will check myself out to see if I actually want to eat.

Words are often more pointed.

"I couldn't help it."

"It's human nature."

"I tried."

These self-pardons act as the green light for the status quo. A go ahead for more of the same. I would rather hear:

"I'm learning more about myself."

"I'm making progress."

"I'm better every day than the day before."

Words have a way of controlling us. I dislike hearing someone say, "I am dying to weigh 120 pounds." I would rather hear, "I would love to weigh 120 pounds."

Words program us. If you ever have a stiff neck, think about who may be giving you "a pain in the neck."

Whether you mouth a phrase like "Oh, my aching back," or "That person galls me," you are giving instructions to your body. Repeated enough and with sufficient emotion, you can manifest physically what you vocalize.

Here are a few more common overweight expressions and suggested substitutions:

- "I'll have to get back on the track."
  (Wait a minute. Eating properly is not that straight and narrow. It's the track to obesity you are on that's straight and narrow. How about just staying off that track?)
- "I just don't have the incentive."

(Are you equating a pound on the scale to your love for a pound of pizza pie? How about asking yourself instead which you love more, "pizza or me?")
- "I want to lose weight but I can't."
(This is a cop-out. It reinforces failure. "I want to be slender and I can." This is reprograming for results.)

Many of my patients turn to the home, office or social problem, leading themselves to seek compensating satisfaction in food. Then they pin the overweight condition on that particular problem.

This is also a cop-out. What they are saying is, "I am not to blame. Other people create these problems. They are to blame for my overweight problem also."

Problems are serious. Insecurity in the job. Friction between two people. Sexual competition. Jealousy. Hate. Fear. Problems can drag you down, if you let them.

Millions of wonderful people are disgusted, rejected, dejected, despaired, depressed, melancholy, down, and confused. The walls of fat they build are no protection; the foods that build the walls are no relief. They wander aimlessly behind the walls, rationalizing, excusing, promising.

Listen to them in the section below.

CRIES IN THE WILDERNESS OF EXCESS

To err is human, to forgive divine.
It's easier said than done.
That is my downfall.
Misery loves company.
Middle-age spread.
I couldn't help it.
It is so difficult.
It's human nature.
What do you expect, perfection?
I tried.
I want.
I wish.
I hope.
I can't.
It's impossible.
If at first you don't succeed,
    try, try, try again.
I don't have enough willpower.
What will be will be.
I might fail.

It really isn't that important.
I don't think.
It's hard to believe.
It's no use. It's hopeless.
I was born with two strikes
    against me.
It's all part of the game.
Fate has dealt me a cruel blow.
I'm fighting it.
I wasn't cut out for success.
It keeps getting harder to lose.
I'm stuck and can't get
    below this weight.
I'm absent-minded.
It's hard to remember,
    easy to forget.
I'm a born loser.
I slipped and slid back.
I should be so lucky. It
    should only happen to me.

It's my destiny.
I can't understand it.
I'm a creature of habit.
I'll stick to the diet.
I'll begin tomorrow.
I'm on a diet.
I'm nervous, irritable,
    depressed, anxious, etc.
I'm a compulsive eater.
I can't accept.
I promise.
New Year's promises.
I'm tired all the time.
I have tired blood.
I have a huge appetite.
I have a sweet tooth.
I can't resist food.
Temptation got the better of me.
What's the use, no one cares.
I'm too old now.
Things are getting worse
    and worse.
You can't trust a soul.
There's just no way out.
I beat my brains out for nothing.
It's easy for you to say.
How can I possibly succeed?
It's for the birds.
I'm on a merry-go-round.
How can I possibly lose
    all this weight?
I am stymied and blocked.
It's hard to get out of a rut.
I'm working at it. I'm
    struggling.
I can't help myself.
I was born to be fat.
Maybe tomorrow.
I keep forgetting.
I'm all mixed up.
I force myself.
I did that but nothing happened.
I will not be able
    to lose weight.
I am not going to succeed.
Everything is against me.
I never get the breaks.
He can but I can't.
I'm a hard luck guy.
It's not in the cards for me.
It just wasn't meant to be.

It's too late. You only
    live once.
Sweets (food) are my downfall.
I can't resist eating when
    food is offered.
I could care less.
I'm not emotional.
I love to eat.
I merely smell food and
    the weight comes back on.
I couldn't refuse or hurt
    her feelings.
I'm emotionally unstrung.
I'm emotional.
My nerves got the better of me.
For some reason or other,
    I stuffed myself, etc.
I'm a weak person. I'm
    not strong willed.
You just don't change overnight.
The weight just happened to creep
    up on me.
I'm getting heavier.
I find it doesn't help.
I don't want to be overweight.
I let down.
God help me. I only hope
    to God.
Is it possible?
No one knows how hard I tried.
I'll fight and lick this problem.
I won't look at food again.
I'll stay away from food.
I feel so guilty and ashamed.
I'm at the end of my rope.
How can anyone possibly
    know or understand?
I'll go on a crash diet.
I was born with a big appetite.
It's hard to break the habit.
I have an inferiority complex.
This weight is getting me down.
I'll lose or drop some weight.
It ain't necessarily so.
I'll watch my weight (diet).
I'm afraid.
It's human nature.
I don't have much confidence,
    desire, determination,
    perseverence, motivation, etc.
For some strange reason . . .

Life has been cruel to me.
Life passed me by.
If I had only done something
    about it a long time ago.
I can only go so far.
I shoulda, (woulda), (coulda)
I'm a victim of circumstances.
I envy her, she is so slim.
It's glandular.
It's hereditary.
I don't have enough time.

I lose and gain—oh well.
My main problem is I eat too
    much.
Now that I've lost weight,
    I can eat again.
Can't I eat good things ever?
It's mind over matter.
I can't write.
So what's the big deal.
It's hard to control myself.
That's the way the cookie crumbles.
I blew it.

Words, these excuses and promises—only words. Can you add a few of your own favorites?

Words relating to a condition or a problem tend to perpetuate that problem.

Words relating to a new condition or a solution tend to create that new condition and bring on a solution.

Here are a few new words to play with:

Understanding
Love
Transformation
Fun
Confidence

What have they to do with losing weight?
You'll see.

"FAT PEOPLE ARE JOLLY PEOPLE!"
(DON'T BELIEVE IT.)

A woman recently wrote to a national columnist deploring the cliché that marriages fall apart when one of the partners gains weight excessively. She pointed out that in their 13 years of marriage she and her husband had each gained about 70 pounds, yet their love life was better than ever. A bonus, she pointed out, was the end of jealousy . . . "Who," she said, "would want either one of them?"

Good humored this writer most certainly is. Valid, no.

Fat people are usually jolly people. Maybe they are—to everyone but themselves.

This has been described very well by one of my patients:

"Fat people are jolly! How many times have you heard that silly, illogical myth repeated? Has some cholesterol conspiracy as ancient as butter perpetrated this Big Fat Lie? Or some mysterious caloric Casa Nostra?

"From Shakespeare's beer-bellied, laughing Falstaff to the modern Mama Cass; from a balloonlike Bacchus with a winsome smile to a rotund red dime store Santa Claus and his Ho!, Ho!, Ho!—always the same phony message.

"Well, I say Ho!, Ho!, Hogwash! It's about time someone exposed this flabby falsity....

"Would you be jolly if you bent over to pick up your canned no-cal lunch and ripped open the seat of your new suit?

"Would you be jolly if, as a kid, you wanted to play baseball and the team captain said, 'Sure you can play—you be the backstop!'

"Would you be jolly if you wore your brand new cocktail dress to a party and overheard a guest saying, 'nice paint job she's got there!'

"Would you be jolly if you sat down in church and the pew tilted?

"Would you be jolly if you went to buy a plane ticket and the smart aleck clerk asked if you wanted a group plan!

"Would you be jolly if you went into a smorgasbord restaurant and the owner burst into tears?

"Would you be jolly if a friend offered you a lift and his seat belts weren't long enough to fit? Or if you did manage to squeeze into one, you arrived at your destination with 'Body by Fisher' stamped just below your navel?

"No my friends, you might laugh with your neighbors. But like me you'd be crying inside."

The big, jolly people are putting up a front.

Deep inside all of that blubber they realize, just as you and I, that even twenty or thirty pounds of excess baggage can be very costly.

They know that obesity can lead to heart attacks, diabetes, circulatory and other physical problems. They know it lessens the chances for successful surgery should it become necessary. They know fat takes years off your life in direct proportion to the amount of excess weight and the time you transport it.

You can't be sincerely jolly about that.

This doesn't mean you can't have fun losing weight. You most certainly can—and will. But you must level with yourself.

You must come from behind the flab, take off your mask, and be perfectly frank with and about yourself.

THE POWER OF MIND OVER CALORIES

Is there someone nearby to help you with a little test? If not, do this test later. Shake hands in the usual way. Then shake hands with your left hands. Feel the difference?

Shaking hands is a perfunctory act with us. It is an automatic motion. We only feel the basic grip.

However, when you shake hands with the left hand, you feel much more—another person's hand in your hand. It is warm. It has texture.

When something is a habit, it requires very little conscious awareness. You can down a couple pieces of pie and never remember the taste afterwards. It's almost like shaking hands with your right hand.

What can you do about eating in order to make the fun more "feelable"?

It stands to reason you will derive more eating pleasure out of something you savour slowly than something you wolf down. This takes concentration. It required concentration for you to shake hands differently—with the left hand. It will require conscious effort on your part to cut a morsel of chicken with your knife and fork, place it in your mouth, then become aware of its flavor as you chew and swallow.

I'm not asking you to forego the chicken. Quite the contrary, I am asking you to enjoy it more by thinking about the pleasure of eating it as you savour its flavor.

I have watched overweight people eat. They don't pay attention to what they are doing. Like it hurts their conscience to know they are eating so they pretend they don't see.

It stands to reason if a person overeats because he seeks pleasure that he doesn't experience in some other way, then he should "live" every mouthful.

Food energy is measured in calories. Some 3,500 calories of food energy, if not expended doing work, can equal one pound of human fat. The usual amount of calories consumed in one day is 2,000 to 3,000, depending on the person's size and degree of activity.

Food pleasure is measured in. . . . Apparently, there is no word for a unit of pleasure. So let's invent one. Let's say it's a "kik." We'll define a kik as the maximum amount of pleasure anyone can derive from eating a medium size apple. We'll make this even more "scientific" and call it a medium size apple of the Red Delicious variety.

Now, I may experience only one-half a kik out of eating such an apple and you may obtain a whole kik out of eating it. It has something to do with how much we enjoy apples. But it also has something to do with how much attention we pay to the apple.

You and I may both enjoy Red Delicious apples equally well. However, I may be concerned about the patients waiting to see me, while you may be thinking about taking the next bite from an untouched part of the apple. I may throw it hurriedly into the garbage while you may have a few more nibbles around the core.

So you derive twice as many kiks from your apple snack as I do.

However, when we are home and the chicken is in front of us, I may forget the office and concentrate on the delicious bird, while you just fill your stomach with it.

So, I may enjoy 33 kiks out of the chicken against your 14. Since the calories are the same, I would derive a higher kik per calorie count than you would.

This kik per calorie is a measure of your enjoyment. The more kiks you experience, the less calories you need.

HOW TO DERIVE MORE PLEASURE FROM THE
FOOD YOU EAT

How do you develop more kiks? It's really very simple. Yet, you may not find yourself doing it that easily or readily. It's like asking you to use your left hand next time you greet someone. It is easy to do, but would you remember?

Any change in our behavior takes concentration. We must keep our mind on it the first few times. Then it becomes automatic, requiring no further special attention.

If I show you how to multiply your kiks per calorie out of everything you eat, you will have to promise me you will do it at every meal for at least a week or more. You will have to exert yourself to remember, but your memory will pay off in two ways:

1. You will be changing your eating habits in that direction and lessening the need for memory later.
2. You will enjoy every meal much more.

Is it a deal?

Then here goes.

You have often heard the term "compulsive eater." You may think anyone who eats more than they should is a compulsive eater. Not true. Impulsive probably, but seldom compulsive.

Compulsive eaters are sick people. How many kiks do you think they derive per calorie? Hardly any. It's an excitement rather than an enjoyment.

Time is the key. Time has to slow down for greater kiks. Here is how you slow your own kik time:

HOW TO: SLOW TIME FOR GREATER EATING ENJOYMENT

- Go into slow motion at the table. Pick up your napkin slowly. Move your hands slowly as you use your spoon, knife and fork.
- Take smaller mouthfuls. Enjoy more mouthfuls per portion.
- Chew more slowly. Extract all the pleasure (kiks) you can from each mouthful.
- Wait before you prepare the next bite until you have swallowed the last. You may wish to set the fork or spoon down between mouthfuls.
- Be aware of what you are doing. You can still carry on a conversation, between, not during mouthfuls.

This is an important step for you to take. It involves more fun eating, not less. It is the first step in winning the battle of mind power over calorie power.

How will you remember?

Here's how: As soon as you finish reading this paragraph, set the book aside and visualize yourself sitting down to your next meal. You know where it will be. See yourself there. See yourself reaching for the napkin to unfold it. See yourself remembering to slow down for greater pleasure the moment you unfold your napkin.

Do this visual exercise now.

These visual (mental) exercises actually program you. You know this as well as I do. You often think about that leftover layer cake in the refrigerator. You picture (imagine) it on the platter. You see just how much is leftover. Now, no amount of self-discipline will help you. You are programed to have a go at it.

Later, I'll describe how to make these visual images even more powerful and effective. Just now all you need do is visualize your napkin triggering a slowdown in your spoon, knife and fork.

TEN SITUATIONS THAT RING A PAVLOV EATING BELL FOR YOU

Do you recall the famous Pavlov experiment with dogs? It is still used as the classic example of the conditioned reflex—or automatic action of the body.

Pavlov, a Russian physiologist whose work dates back nearly a century ago, connected devices to the dogs to measure the flow of saliva in their mouth. Every time he fed the dogs, he rang a bell. Soon, he merely had to ring a bell and the saliva would flow.

How many have similar "bells" or conditioned reflexes? The answer is—all of us do.

Going to the movies may sound a bell for popcorn. An outing at the beach may sound a bell for a hot dog or frankfurter. A television commercial may ring your urge for a beer. Or just sitting down to watch television may sound the bell for potato chips.

There are many subtle bells which make your saliva flow or your hunger symptoms felt. Here are some to which you may be responding:

- Being in the kitchen.
- Sitting at the dining table.
- Playing cards.
- Having a cup of coffee or tea.
- Shopping.
- Talking on the phone.
- Knowing what time it is.
- Being tired.
- Being annoyed, frustrated, lonely or similar emotion.
- Being party to good news, festivity, social activity.
- Etc., etc.

Betty checked her "bells." She found that she was still "wired" to the two coffee breaks she used to take when working. Now a housewife, the urge to indulge in a hot cup or two and to go with it, a danish or two, came like clockwork at 10:00 a.m. and at 3:00 p.m.

George, an assistant manager in a bowling establishment, enjoyed talking about his experiences in the army. Invariably, this led to a few beers, plus appropriate accoutrements.

Laurel liked to tell her friends to hold the wire while she poured a cup of hot coffee. With the cup came a plate of glazed doughnuts. Her Pavlov bell was "wired" to ring with the telephone bell.

Are you "wired" for food? Is your time hunger being short-circuited by mental reflexes or conditionings that claim to be hunger? If so, what can you do about it?

In a moment I shall explain how to identify and "de-bug" what is triggering false hunger for you. Then be ready for some changes in your life.

L.C. overate because she was lonely when her husband left on frequent business trips. L.C.'s husband promised her a new wardrobe if she lost 15 pounds. It required ten weeks. The difference was so pronounced—more youthful coloring, more enthusiasm, a bubbly, outgoing personality—that he bought her a mink coat, too. Even more important, he was so proud of her, they hired a "live-in" baby sitter and he took L.C. with him on his business trips.

When a business executive does some thinking about conditioned eating and then deconditions herself, the whole business feels it. H.K., 53, was tired, grouchy, and short tempered. In 17 weeks she shed 19 pounds. Dizzy spells, hot flashes, high blood pressure and aching legs disappeared. She was no longer short with employees. Business associates complimented her slim figure and noticed how well she looked. Needless to say, her spirits soared and so did business.

Visualize a person who rarely talks, wears heavy glasses, bites her nails, slumps over due to her 6'2" height, and has 172 pounds of rather odorous body.

Now see that person as smiling, standing erect, self-confident, long polished nails, contact lenses, hygienic in her appearance, and stylish in her dress.

Did I make a miracle? No, she did. And you can imagine what it did for her students. K.S. was a school teacher. And for her husband? At 145 and still descending, her weight was just one symptom of a woman who had found herself.

HOW TO "DE-BUG" YOUR FALSE HUNGER BELLS

Often you think about your emotions, discover what is "bugging" your appetite, "de-bug" it, and just when you think you have the answer, along comes another problem to "bug" your appetite all over again.

> Take L.E., a married woman, 220 pounds, 5'7", age 41, working as an instrument calibrator. Her daughter was chronically ill. Her son sentenced to prison. When she realized that overeating was her way of coping with these problems, she lost weight steadily. Then her husband became involved in a court custody battle over children by a former marriage and she hit the refrigerator, and 200 pounds, again.
> The solution is to continue with self-analysis. Then program yourself against capitulating to trouble via the kitchen.

Whenever you are being "bugged," you must locate the device. The same is true for "appetite bugging." What is your favorite snack time? When do you enjoy hitting the refrigerator or the lunch counter for that extra bite or ten?

When does your Pavlov bell ring? You may not know at this very moment. But in 24 hours you can have your sights on the various "triggers." In 48 hours you can have confirmations of your suspicions. And in 72 hours you can know for sure.

Re-examine the above list for clues. Think about yourself and when you desire to eat. Keep a diary of every drink or mouthful. Include what you were doing or thinking at the moment.

The pattern should become apparent. And you are then ready to pull out the unwanted wires.

Some bell ringers that can work for you

Meanwhile, here are a few things you can do that will help to anticipate what lies ahead. They are common Pavlov bells which work on most of us.

1. The spots where you usually eat or snack trigger memories. The fewer such spots, the fewer such memories. Manage to eat in as few places as possible. If you always eat at home, arrange to eat only at one particular table, using one special place and placemat.
2. Lower the volume of your television set during commercials, regardless of what is being sold. Then pick up a good book (this one?) and enjoy it for a few minutes.
3. Avoid the kitchen, except for regular meals or their preparation. If you must, keep a pitcher of ice water or pot of hot, decaffeinated coffee elsewhere to refrain from pulling that oldie on yourself.

4. If there is tension in the house, postpone eating until the situation is under control.

5. Chew gum (sugarless variety) while preparing meals and cleaning the kitchen.

These are examples of how to "handle" bells. They are largely avoidance measures and help to avoid the exact circumstances that ring the phony appetite bell.

Later, we will learn how to disconnect the phony bells altogether, dismantle them, and toss them into the garbage can.

Then you will begin to create your own valid hunger bells that ring only *when your body needs food.*

THE MIRACLE RULE OF TWO—ADDING
TO REGULAR EATING TIMES

Time marches on.

When appetite bells are harnessed to the hands of the clock, the pointer on the scale moves too.

How do you cope with that type bell? Well, I promised you that aimless, tedious discipline and willpower don't make for a fun way of slenderizing. Therefore, I won't ask you to abstain from eating during those extra times that habit has created.

Instead, I do ask you to eat during those times. But let's you and I fool the Pavlov bell-ringer. Let's save part of our meals for the times when he rings that bell.

In other words, let's add two feedings to the number of times we are used to eating. If you only eat two meals a day, the rule of two states you can now enjoy eating four times a day. Not four meals, four times. It is the same two meals as before; however, you now eat them in two installments.

If you eat three meals a day, eat five times a day.

If you eat four meals a day, eat six times a day.

Here's how you can split breakfast into two installments, if that is one of the meals you need to divide in order to place part of it on a Pavlov bell.

7:00 a.m.	*10:00 a.m.*
Orange Juice	Scrambled Eggs
Coffee (decaffeinated)	Coffee (decaffeinated)
	or non-fat milk

If your Pavlov appetite bell rings in mid-afternoon, then lunch will be the meal that is eaten at two sittings. Lunches can be split similar to this:

Noon	*3:00 p.m.*
Consommé	Hamburger Steak, onions
Cole Slaw	Coffee (decaffeinated)
Tea with lemon	or low calorie beverage

If you have split both breakfast and lunch, then have your dinner at one sitting. However, if only one of these meals have been enjoyed at two sittings, then dinner should be split similar to this:

7:00 p.m.	*11:00 p.m.*
Pork Chops	Maple Cream Dessert
Spinach	Coffee (decaffeinated)
Salad	or non-fat milk
Coffee (decaffeinated)	

There is evidence we do more than fool the Pavlov bells by this maneuver. Doctors often recommend frequent, smaller meals. This avoids overloading the body's fuel supply. When you eat more than the body requires over the next few hours, the permanent storage facilities are brought into action to handle the surplus.

Where are your permanent storage facilities—your buttocks, hips, thighs, stomach, neck, arms. See the picture?

25 TIPS TO MAKE LIFE EASIER AS YOU SLIM DOWN

The "rule of two" about splitting meals is something you need not do now. It's a tip you may find helpful, now or later.

Few of my patients want to ease into that shift in eating habits so soon. That's fine with me. I want to make the plan available to you, to implement whenever useful.

If not, hold it in abeyance.

Here are additional tips to make life easier while you shift into a healthier manner of eating and a thinking-about-yourself program.

Again, these are not for immediate application. You would drive your family and yourself out of their mind.

I offer them as optional tools to use if they can be helpful.

Most are aimed at removing moments when everything is

perfect for a Pavlov bell to ring. Why subject yourself to temptation? Why trigger false appetites unnecessarily?

Here goes:

- Concentrate on eating as you eat. Don't watch television, play cards, or talk on the phone while eating. Don't read or perform tasks.
- Use the same placemats or distinctly colored table cloth and napkins for every meal, wherever possible.
- Shop for food soon after the largest meal of the day. Definitely avoid shopping when hungry.
- Make a shopping list of high protein, low fat/carbohydrate foods (see next chapter) and don't allow sweet and starchy supermarket sights move you.
- Leftover salads, meats, etc. make great snacks. Avoid buying snack foods.
- Educate your table mates about your choice of nourishing foods; if they balk, let them fend for themselves.
- Clear plates directly into the garbage pail to avoid making yourself one.
- Place only enough food on the table for average single portions. Any leftovers can be used as snacks later.
- Encourage harmony at the table. Postpone discussion of problems and debatable issues until after the meal is finished.
- Clean the kitchen of all high calorie condiments, high fat salad dressings, candy, potato chips, marshmallows, frozen cake and ice cream, etc. Give them to someone you don't like.
- Use smaller dinner plates, if available. Spread the food. Use parsley, lettuce beds and other esthetic means to dress the plate.
- Schedule meals at regular times.
- Vary your menus. There are thousands of meals possible with many high protein foods available and several ways to prepare them.
- Develop a million dollar taste. Be a gourmet. Know what good is.
- Develop an eagle eye for fats and carbohydrates. Learn how to spot them in recipes and develop ways to circumvent them. (I'll be helping you with this in the chapters ahead.)
- Place your knife and fork, or spoon on the plate from time to time as an aid to slowing your eating pace.
- Review from time to time the averse consequences of overeating, how excessive weight shortens life, how fat slows you down on your job, and in your social activities.
- Reward yourself when you lose weight. Buy a new dress, outfit, shirt, suit. Go to a show.
- Talk about your weight reducing activities only with those likely to be in sympathy with what you are doing. Don't expect support from those more likely to give you "flack."

- Make a graph of your weight progress. Chart your present weight on the left. Make entries once or twice a week. Note your goal (don't give a date). Post the graph in a conspicuous place, such as your refrigerator door.
- Become more active physically. Walk up a few flights of stairs instead of riding the elevator. Don't fret about parking a distance from your job or shopping. Do exercises in spare moments.
- Read labels on cans and packages. Avoid preservatives and processed foods whenever possible. Look for the fresh and natural.
- Relax and visualize yourself reaching your weight goal. See yourself attractive, admired and slim. Do this at least a minute each day.
- Think about yourself. Take a bird's-eye view of your life. Especially your childhood, your young adulthood, your love life, your fears, anxieties, your hopes, your problems. How do these views affect your appetite, your eating habits?
- Keep pad and pen handy to jot down thoughts about yourself, ideas, conclusions, theories, insight. Record your "crutches," rationalizations, problems, situations, feelings and emotions.

These are the tools to help do. It is wiser to think in terms of things to do rather than things not to do.

It is hard not to do something. Remembering what you are not supposed to do keeps the unwanted action in your mind. ("I am off sweets . . . sweets . . . sweets.") Can't you just see the built-in failure factor?

It is much easier to remember to do something. ("I can eat all the lean hamburger steak I need to satisfy me.") Are not the odds very much against this person turning to sweets? So here we have a high success factor.

Read the 25 tips again. Check off those you plan to use now. Note that many have to do with food shopping and home eating patterns. These are good areas in which to begin.

In the next chapter we discuss food. As you read details of the food program, let your mind dwell on the delicious meats, fish, poultry and other highly nutritious foods you'll soon enjoy. Now dismiss from your mind the sweets, starches and empty calorie "foods"—if one can call them that—which are your body's enemy. Mark them well—but drop them from your consciousness.

Anticipate the guilt-free fun you will now experience eating properly.

Expect a glorious change in your looks and your life to begin.

The Meat of Chapter 2

Watch your language. Drop failure words and "cop-outs." Adopt positive words that program you for success.

Turn on your awareness about food. Step up your enjoyment factor. Derive more "kiks" out of everything you eat. "Live" every wonderful mouthful.

Go into slow motion while you eat. Make it last. No one gets maximum enjoyment out of quickie anything.

Identify the appetite bells in your home, office and environment. Minimize them by avoiding the kitchen, etc.

Split some meals, adding two sittings to your eating day without increasing quantity.

See how quickly you can act on all 25 tips—and tip the scales in favor of the slender you.

3

HOW TO EAT CORRECTLY FOR A FULL BELLY
AND A SLENDER PROFILE

Appetizer for Chapter 3

Now we will talk about food. As you know food is not exactly my favorite subject.

You are.

Yet there are right foods and wrong foods. You can fill your belly with the non-fattening foods and still lose weight.

You may take just a nibble or two of the fattening foods now and then and "blow it."

This is an eating program, not a non-eating program. Here is how to enjoy good eating—with some of my very favorite recipes thrown in at no extra charge.

I hesitate to take your valuable time now to discuss food.

Food is a symptom not a reason for your overweight problem. I would rather we talk about reasons than symptoms, just so we don't eat while we talk.

I would rather we...

- TAKE TIME TO THINK
   It is the source of power.
- TAKE TIME TO PLAY
   It is the secret of perpetual youth.
- TAKE TIME TO READ
   It is the fountain of wisdom.

- TAKE TIME TO LOVE AND BE LOVED
  It is a God-given privilege.
- TAKE TIME TO BE FRIENDLY
  It is the road to happiness.
- TAKE TIME TO LAUGH
  It is the music of the soul.
- TAKE TIME TO GIVE
  It is too short a day to be selfish.
- TAKE TIME TO WORK
  It is the price of success.
- TAKE TIME TO PRAY
  It is the greatest power on earth.

I put powerful material such as this on my office bulletin board; also clippings from magazines, newspapers, etc. I can't quote the source of this material so I cannot give credit where certainly much credit is due.

It is especially great for a weight-loss program. Not only does it omit "TAKE TIME TO EAT," it also places emphasis on the more important aspects of life.

Before we talk about food, remember to place your priorities accordingly—think, play, read, love, befriend, laugh, give, work, pray.

And did you notice which came first?

FILL YOUR BELLY WITH THESE FOODS
AND YOU CANNOT GO WRONG

I have mentioned briefly how fats and carbohydrates are your enemies. They supply more energy than one can use, so you store them. Like a camel prepared for dry days ahead, you acquire mounds of stored-up material. The only difference is, with you the "dry" days never come: there is always more food around than the energy output requires. So your mounds grow.

Many overweight people are undernourished. They are so hung up on sweets and starches, they build mounds of fat while they starve their bones, tissues, blood, and vital organs of replacement proteins, minerals, and other critically needed nutrients.

Fill your belly with protein foods and high mineral and vitamin content foods, instead of fats and carbohydrates, and watch the fat melt away as your posture improves, your profile slims, and your gait quickens.

"I was so overjoyed to lie in the tub and not feel my body hemmed in on both sides. I now fit in my bathtub. And, standing, I can see my knees."

The comments are those of a formerly fat woman who somehow managed to operate a computer despite her 294 pounds. She had no sexual relations with her husband for two years. A 30-pound drop in her weight and she fit the tub. A 50-pound drop brought her sex. Then she thought she had it made and left the program. She returned within six months, ready for additional reprograming.

Another case—would you believe a 20-year old girl looked like a 50-year old spinster? That's what about 50 excess pounds did for L.D., whose 178 pounds kept her from most jobs except babysitting. Her hair was actually turning gray and her old-fashioned clothes and unkempt appearance couldn't have been improved upon by a Hollywood make-up artist.

In one year's time she lost 30 years in her appearance. She became a beautiful young girl and began dating the best looking men. "I'm having a great time and feel fantastic." She didn't have to tell me, I could see it. She enrolled in school to become a nurse.

Patients are proud when they lose weight. Very often I become so involved with their progress that I share their pride with them. I'll never forget little O.C. She was 17 and weighed 190. She actually never experienced and enjoyed normal weight, having just gained as she grew, and grew as she gained. At 5'2" she agreed it was necessary to lose at least 50 pounds.

Since it's usually tough shedding for a teenager, I had misgivings, but she was highly motivated. The following dates and weights are extracted from the records:

April 6, 1973—190
May 18, 1973—159
June 15, 1973—146
June 29, 1973—144
July 27, 1973—138

She rushed to the scale each time she came in; told everyone how much she lost; showed off her new dental assistant uniform; and elevated us all with her excitement and enthusiasm.

Although weight loss is understandably important, this young teenager will better comprehend her miracle in the years ahead as she realizes more and more the importance of self-understanding and self-discovery.

"Doctor, should I eat the white chicken meat or dark?"

"Do I broil the lobster or boil it?"

"Which cut of beef is better—the sirloin or tenderloin?"

"Are frogs legs fish or meat?"

"Which are lower in calories, squab or guinea hen?"

I have one standard answer for such questions: "It doesn't matter."

Perhaps it does matter. But so slightly, it doesn't matter.

Once you make the switch to protein living, the details are lost in the immensity of the changes you'll notice. Why quibble about how many calories in a rib chop versus a loin chop, when chops permit you to slim whereas the spaghetti prevents you from slimming?

Let's take a bird's-eye view of the *right* foods. Then we'll descend into more and more details.

First—here are your best foods:

Beef	Seafood
Veal	Salad
Lamb	Leafy Vegetables
Poultry	Eggs
Fish	Some Cheeses

I could stop here and many of you would be able to proceed on your own. But I can hear the questions already: What cuts? How about organ meats? Can I use spices? Which are the best vegetables? What about fruits? Dressings? Beverages? Desserts?

So let's come down from that bird's-eye view and take in more of the details you need to know.

HOW TO: HIGH PROTEIN, LOW FAT, LOW CARBOHYDRATE FOODS FOR MIRACLE WEIGHT (AND FAT) LOSS PROGRAM

MEAT   Beef, veal and lamb. All cuts including stew, chops, roasts, steaks, and organs. Ground lean meat for patties. Lean pork only, such as well done chops. Remove all visible fat from meats. Then broil, boil, roast or barbeque.

POULTRY   Chicken, turkey, squab, Cornish hen. Avoid poultry skin where fat is usually concentrated. No duck or goose.

FISH   All fresh and salt water varieties including tuna, salmon, cod, halibut, flounder, bass, trout. Avoid prepared fish cakes or fish fries containing bread crumbs or other wheat filling or coating.

SEAFOOD   Lobster, clams, crabs, shrimp, oysters, mussels, crayfish, etc.

SALAD   All types of lettuce, cabbage and greens plus scallions, radishes, celery, green peppers, small tomato, and other raw vegetables from the list below. Low calorie (diet) dressing only, except your own dressing made with one part safflower oil, three parts vinegar, economically applied. Fennel, pepper and other spices may be used.

VEGE-
TABLES   Asparagus, beet greens (no beets), broccoli, cabbage, carrots, cauliflower, celery, chard, chicory, Chinese cabbage, collard, cucumber, endive, escarole, kale, kohlrabi, leek, mushrooms, mustard greens, onions, peppers, pickles (dill), pimentos, radishes, rhubarb, spinach, turnip, squash (green), string beans, watercress.

CHEESE   Low fat cheeses such as American, Camembert, Cheddar, Cottage, Edam, Farmers, Gouda, Gruyere, Mozzarella, Muenster, Parmesan, Pot, Provolone, Ricotta, Romano, Swiss, Tilsiter.

EGGS   Any style (no butter or oil, use Teflon coated pan or Panstick, Pam, etc.).

FRUIT   ONCE A DAY. Preferred fruits are grapefruit (½), cantaloupe, honeydew or casaba melon, peach, pear, plum, strawberries, blackberries, gooseberries (all berry portions are to be small), watermelon (small wedge). Fresh fruit is preferred. If canned, use water or natural juice pack (not sugar syrup).

BEVER-
AGES   Water, decaffeinated coffee (black), weak tea (lemon permitted), buttermilk or non-fat milk (two glasses daily limit), tomato juice (8-ounce daily limit), low calorie soft drinks (3 or less calories per can, limit: 2 cans per day). IMPORTANT: *Drink eight full glasses of liquid a day.* Coffee lovers should switch to decaffeinated. It reduces nervousness, provides less gastric stimulation, and cuts up-and-down false hunger cycles.

QUAN-
TITY   Eat all you need to satisfy true hunger. If weight reaches a plateau, first decrease fruit intake, followed by a limitation of vegetables. Be sure the remaining fruits and vegetables are the lowest calorie varieties.

HOW TO MARSHAL YOUR DEFENSES
AGAINST FATS AND CARBOHYDRATES

This is a weight (and fat) loss program. When you reach your desired goal, you continue onto the weight maintenance program.

The maintenance program is very dissimilar to a standard "starvation" diet. It is so permissive you wonder why you don't regain poundage. But you don't. The secret is in the low level of fats and carbohydrates compared to your intake before you started on the program.

So it boils down to keeping a wary eye open and an educated mouth closed for fats and carbohydrates.

Would you think there is any fat or carbohydrate in frankfurters? Indeed, there is. Recently, there was a national expose on how much fat and filler is actually in these American favorites. I say avoid them.

Read the small print on most bologna, salami, sausage and other prepared meats. You'll see preservatives and chemicals listed which make them a poor choice compared to fresh meats. In most fresh meats the fat is visible and can be cut away by your fat-militant knife.

FOODS THAT ARE "YES, YES"
AND THOSE THAT ARE "NO, NO"

Let's drop even lower from that bird's-eye view so we can read some of the labels in your kitchen.

I want to give the nod specifically to certain items we see there so that there is no doubt in your mind you can use them in this slenderizing program.

On the other hand, I want you to be absolutely sure about not using other items. The criteria are, of course, fats and carbohydrates.

First: *Yes, Yes*

- Clear broth and bouillon (like clam, chicken, beef, etc.).
- Soups without fat or starchy thickeners.
- Horseradish, mustard, onion (powder or dried flakes), catsup.

- Artificial sweeteners (e.g. saccharin), salt substitues.
- Soy sauce, A-1 sauce, L'Escoffier sauce, etc.
- All seasonings, spices and condiments.

This list is not complete. I say "yes, yes" to many items brought to my attention just so I see they are relatively free of fats and carbohydrates.

You do likewise. Check out questionable items with my eyes. Now for: *No! No!*

- Alcoholic beverages including beer and wine, until you are ready for your maintenance program.
- Duck, goose, bacon, pork (except lean chops), hot dogs, smoked meats, fat in any meat, sausage, bologna and similar cold cut meats. Only small portions of liver.
- Fruits such as avocado, bananas, cherries, dates, dried fruits, fruits canned in syrup, grapes, raisins, apricots, apples, oranges and orange juice—other specified fruits are permitted on a one-portion-per-day basis.
- Baked goods such as bread (one slice per day of whole, freshly ground grain permitted if weight loss is at an acceptable rate), biscuits, cake, cereals (hot or cold), cookies, crackers, doughnuts, muffins, pancakes, pies, pretzels, rolls, spaghetti and other pastas, waffles.
- Butter, creams (sweet or sour), cream cheese, margarine, mayonnaise, milk (whole or evaporated), yogurt, sauces made with flour or butter.
- Candy, chocolate, cocoa, coconut, dessert toppings, honey, ices, sherbets, ice cream, sugar, syrup, jam, jelly, marmalade, similar snack foods.
- Fried foods, french fries, potatoes, popcorn, potato chips.
- Smoked fish, sardines.
- Corn, rice, cornstarch.
- Starchy vegetables like peas, lima beans, sweet potatoes.
- Nuts, oils, peanuts, peanut butter.
- Salt, salad dressings (except safflower oil and vinegar or low-calorie preparations).
- Soft drinks (except low calorie type), cream soups, gravy.

HOW TO REDUCE FAT CONTENT IN FOOD, COOKING, AND YOU

You can put a big "C" or a big "F" opposite each of the "No! No!" items, flagging them as carbohydrate or fat.

Carbohydrates are easy to spot. They are the sweets and starches. Alcohol turns to carbohydrate. But basically, flour and sugar are the two worst offenders. Some vegetables are starchy, such as beets, and so are most grains, such as corn and rice. All fruits contain carbohydrate, some more than others. Therefore, only one piece or portion is allowed per day until you reach your goal and go on the maintenance program.

Fats are more secretive than carbohydrates. They know how to hide. They hide in the veins of meat, in the butter fat of cheese, in the oil of nuts.

Here are several tips to spot fats, both in solid and oil form, so you can minimize them and make the program work even more efficiently for you.

HOW TO: FOOD PREPARATION FOR
MINIMIZING FATS AND CARBOHYDRATES

- Favor leaner meats. Cut all visible fat from meat before cooking. Hamburger is often marked "extra lean." This usually contains less than 10 percent fat and is preferred.
- Remove the skin from poultry when serving yourself. White meat has less fat than dark, but the difference does not warrant your lessened enjoyment if you prefer dark.
- Select low fat types of cottage cheese, and other low fat cheeses made from skim (non-fat) milk.
- Use water-packed canned fish. If only oil-packed is available, rinse off the oil before using.
- Use milk products with milk fat removed—skim milk and skim milk powder are good, usable examples. Plain, low fat yogurt is permitted in small amounts.
- Substitute for rich creams and toppings (used in desserts and dips at parties) the low calorie milk products such as whipped evaporated skim milk, whipped cottage cheese or yogurt, or flavored skim milk powder.
- Broil for lowest residual fat in cooked meats. Brown or render such meats as stews and roasts and pour off fat. Stews can be cooked a half day early, cooled, then the solid fat removed.
- If you must fry, use a Teflon pan, Panstick, or Pam. Avoid recipes with butter or margarine. If you wish, use artificial butter flavor.
- Use natural juice gravies only, cooling first and separating the fat.
- Don't baste roasts with fatty cooking liquids. Use a special spoon that separates natural juice. Or use BBQ bastes or tomato juice with herbs. Wine is a permissible baste since alcohol evaporates. Bastes for fish might include lemon juice (with chopped parsley), clam juice, skim milk.

KNOW THE CHANGES YOU MUST MAKE,
THEN "THINKING" MAKES IT EASY

Harriet, 29, was a big, loud, buxom blonde in the classic sense. Today, she is no longer as big, as buxom, or quite as loud or blonde. She owed her classic stature to such classic delicacies as hot dogs and hamburgers. But let her tell you . . .

"I recently began wondering about my eating habits—why, for instance, is a hamburger in a paper bag nearly irresistible to me? And why do I prefer to eat at hot dog stands and drive-ins?

"I believe my hamburger-in-a-bag thing is conditioning—an acquired taste. It is attractive because someone cooked it for me, such as at home when mother always packed my lunch or fixed my dinner. All I had to do was eat and enjoy. No fuss, no muss. It also means love. Mother takes care of me because she loves me.

"Lately, however, I have been cooking more meals at home. I find it is not all that difficult if you just have the correct attitude and don't make it a more difficult chore than it really is.

"I am gaining confidence slowly, as a result of this program. The toning down of my hair color is a case in point. I no longer feel the need to be a 'big blond.' I'm sure my natural color will do nicely, in fact I like it this way.

"I also don't feel the need to entertain everyone by being funny all the time. I still think a sense of humor is important and it is part of me, but I don't feel I must be 'turned on' with people I'm not comfortable with. I find I am comfortable in most situations now.

"There is much to be improved upon but I am making good progress."

Harriet has come a long way since she analyzed her craving for that bag of hamburgers or frankfurters. She's a poised, confident, slender person.

When you begin to know, it begins to show.

Of course, the first thing you have to know is which foods are causing the problem.

Those foods are fats and carbohydrates.

I am not advocating an extreme or unbalanced intake. I openly oppose an all protein diet or an all protein and fat diet. There are too many risks involved with eliminating all carbohydrates, such as low blood sugar and excessive ketones or acid in the system.

Some fat is necessary for the body. In fact, fats are an essential building material for nerve and brain tissue and for cushioning vital organs such as the kidney, heart and liver. Also, certain fats are essential for glandular health, especially the prostate glands in men. Fat lubricates joints, skin, and scalp.

Safflower oil is a valuable fat for the body and is recommended as part of your salad dressing. Only small quantities are needed. You know how only a small amount of oil is necessary to lubricate a machine. Your body can easily survive on a teaspoon of oil.

The penalty calorie-wise for using more fat than you need comes high. A gram of any other food is equal to four calories. But a gram of fat produces nine calories—more than twice as much.

So here is what you know:

* You know you must avoid oils and fatty foods.
* You know you must devise low fat cookery.
* You know you must eliminate the butter and margarine "habit."
* You know you must favor proteins in your marketing and menus. This means meat, poultry, fish, eggs, cheese.
* You know you must eat only certain vegetables that are more leafy and less starchy in character.
* You know you must decrease your fruit intake to one portion per day.
* You know you must avoid liquor, also sweet sodas but can enjoy tea, coffee, and low calorie sodas.

BECOME VERSATILE IN PREPARING YOUR
FAVORITE PROTEIN FOODS

Can you smell a delicious aroma coming from the kitchen.
It is mushrooms cooking.

Mushrooms happen to be one of my favorite foods. They are also low in calories, low in carbohydrates, high in nourishment and taste satisfaction—at least to me.

I have some mushrooms baking right now. When through they will taste similar to roast peanuts. If you want an innocent snack, this is a good bet. Here's how you go about it.

Take canned button mushrooms, drain off the liquid, and spread the mushrooms evenly on an aluminum foil tray or cookie tin. Sprinkle them with a salt substitute. Then bake in a slow oven

(250° F.) for about an hour. Check and remove when the mushrooms are brown and thoroughly dry.

I enjoy mushroom sauce over beef, hard boiled eggs, chicken, and fish. I take firm white mushrooms (1 cup) and, after washing them, slice them lengthwise so each slice includes cap and stem. Then I mix them in a heavy saucepan with instant chicken broth mix (1 envelope), and a little water (¼ cup). Cover the saucepan and cook five minutes. Then stir in two tablespoons of nonfat dry milk powder. You now have a magic sauce in which to heat that leftover meat and turn it into an instant feast.

I make mushroom casseroles, mushroom salads, and mushroom soups.

What are some of your favorite foods? Steak? Chicken? There are any number of ways to cook, season, and serve steak. If you learn to use them, you can keep steak high on your list of taste pleasures. The same with chicken and most other food.

High protein dining is fun.

Become an innovator and experimenter. Expand your dining horizons into the gourmet world of new taste thrills.

25 "DISCOVERY" RECIPES FOR ELEGANT DINING WHILE YOU SHED WEIGHT

Gumbos, curries, and fondues.

Deviled this, sauteed that, and fascinating dishes "jardiniere," "provencale," or "marengo."

Sound complicated? Like too much trouble? Not so. Here are 25 easy recipes using ordinary ingredients but producing extraordinary dining pleasure.

They are all program-oriented. You know what that means—carbohydrate and fat content is at a minimum, nutrition is at a maximum. I didn't originate them and don't know who did. They have probably evolved since their original versions. For example, butter has been eliminated, or something substituted for flour or bread crumbs.

These recipes for your use now include two appetizers, four soups, seven entrees, three vegetables or salads, seven desserts, and two party dips.

I told you we're going to have fun.

HOW TO: RECIPES FOR 25 DELICIOUS DISHES
FOR YOUR MIRACLE WEIGHT (AND FAT) LOSS PROGRAM*

SOUPS

Vegetable Quickie (For 2)

¼ C Shredded cabbage	2½ C Water
¼ C Onion, chopped	2 Beef bouillon cubes
½ C Diced carrots	¼-½ t Salt
½ C Celery and leaves	3 Peppercorns
1 Bay leaf (remove	¼ t Thyme
before serving)	1 Sprig parsley, cut up
1 C Tomato juice	

Combine all ingredients and simmer on low heat for 1 hour.

Vegetable Chicken (For 3)

1 lb. Chicken wings	2 Sprigs parsley
and backs	½ C Celery leaves
3½ C Water	1 Bay leaf
3-4 Carrots, halved	1/8 t Marjoram, thyme,
2 Stalks green onion,	and tarragon
cut into pieces	1 t Salt

Place all ingredients in large heavy saucepan. Cover and bring to boil. Lower heat to simmer for 2 or more hours. Strain and refrigerate. Skim off fat before reheating. Sprinkle with bits of green onion and serve.

Balkan Soup (For 4)

1¼ C Buttermilk	Pinch of dried
2 C Yogurt (plain)	marjoram, dill
1 Hard-boiled egg, chopped	2 Sprigs Chinese or
½ Large cucumber, diced	regular parsley,
¼ C Ice water	chopped

Mix all ingredients together by hand or in blender or mixer. Refrigerate. Sprinkle chopped chives in each bowl at serving time.

---

*Abbreviations: C = Cup
t = Teaspoon
T = Tablespoon
Salt = Use a substitute whenever possible

Egg-Drop Soup Occidental

Bring to simmer canned chicken soup (or home-made). Drop in one raw egg per person and let cook for about 2 minutes. Sprinkle with chopped chives and serve.

APPETIZERS

Mushrooms Camelot (For 4-5)

1 Package of Mushrooms	¼ t Soy sauce
1 T Celery, chopped	2 T Pinenuts
3 T Bleu cheese	Olives, parsley for
Dash of curry, nutmeg	garnish

Wash and dry mushrooms. Cut off stems. Blend together all other ingredients and fill mushroom caps. Serve cold, garnished with parsley and sliced olives.

Celery Stuffed with Roquefort

Clean celery. Use long flat stalks with leaves. Mash Roquefort cheese with fork and mix well with cottage cheese until thick mixture results. Mix in chopped celery leaves to taste and heap up on celery sticks.

ENTREES

Steak Surabaya (For 1)

8 Oz. Sirloin steak	Freshly ground pepper
1½ T Warmed brandy	to taste

Cut off all fat and rub thoroughly with pepper on both sides. Broil. Serve immediately, igniting the brandy. (This causes alcohol and last vestiges of fat to be removed.)

Roast Chicken Sauterne (For 4)

1 4-lb. Chicken	1 t Paprika
1 Clove garlic	3/4 C Dry Sauterne
½ Small lemon,	Gooseberries
cut into wedges	

Rub chicken thoroughly with garlic, lemon wedges, paprika, salt and freshly ground pepper. Stuff with gooseberries. Roast at 325° until done (about 1 hour), basting with wine. Serve with pan juices (skimmed of all fat) and with the gooseberries.

Beef Tartar (For 3)

1 lb. Finely ground beef (no fat)	1 Garlic cube, minced or pressed
1 Egg	Salt, pepper to taste
¼ t Freshly squeezed ginger	

Mix ginger and garlic into meat, form into patties. Flatten with large spoon and place raw egg yolk in indentation. Decorate with capers or chia seeds.

Algerian Shortribs (For 4)

2 lbs. Beef shortribs	1/8 t Salt, cumin, cinnamon
1 Medium onion	3-4 Peppercorns

Cover meat with water; sprinkle with salt and let soak for 15 minutes. Drain, pat dry, and rub with seasonings. In heavy pan brown meat and sliced onions. Drain off all fat. Lower heat, cover pan and cook at simmer until tender.

West Coast Spinach (For 4)

½ lb. Beef, calves, or chicken liver	5-6 Mushrooms, washed, sliced
2 Packages frozen spinach, defrosted	1 Small onion
	2 Raw eggs

Cut up livers into small slices (chill or partly freeze to make it easier to slice). Saute in small amount of oil with sliced onion and sliced mushrooms. Add other ingredients and stir. Heat thoroughly. Season with salt and pepper. Sprinkle paprika on top and serve.

Mushroom Fillets (For 4)

2 lbs. Flounder or Haddock fillets	1 T Vinegar
1 Small minced onion	3 Fresh mushrooms
Lemon wedges	Pinch of dill, thyme, basil
2 Sprigs parsley	Paprika
	Salad oil

Rub fillet with a little oil, paprika. Place under broiler with vinegar in pan. Broil on one side until fillets flake easily, but are still moist. Meanwhile, saute mushrooms and onions in as little oil as possible. Sprinkle with herbs. Place fillets on serving platter. Top with mushrooms and onions and garnish with parsley and lemon wedges.

Meat Loaf (For 4)

1 lb. Lean chopped beef
1 Small Green pepper,
    finely chopped
1 Small Carrot, grated
1 Small Onion, chopped

1 Clove Garlic
½ C Skimmed milk
2 T Dry red wine
1/8 t Oregano, thyme

In Teflon saucepan, lightly cook the vegetables. Add all other ingredients and mix thoroughly. Place in loaf pan and cook 45 minutes in medium oven.

VEGETABLES

Cauliflower with Pinenuts (For 3)

1 Large Cauliflower
2½ t Soy flour
1/8 t Dried marjoram or
    thyme

1 C Skim milk
1 Doz. Pinenuts
Dash of Worcestershire
    sauce

Prepare cauliflower by cutting flowerets from stalk and thinly slicing stalk into bite-size pieces. Wash and cook in a little water until tender. Drain, leaving liquid in saucepan. To this add soy flour and blend well over low heat. Add milk, salt and pepper to taste and herbs. Stir until thickened, add nuts, heat and serve over cauliflower.

Italian Green Beans (For 3)

1 Pkg. Frozen Italian
    green beans
1 Strip Lean bacon, cooked
    and crumbled
1 Small Tomato, cut up
Dash Oregano

1 Small Clove garlic,
    minced
Salt, pepper to taste
1 T green onion, finely
    sliced
1 T green pepper, chopped

Saute bacon and remove. Pour off fat. Now slightly brown onions, green pepper and garlic in same saucepan. Add beans, tomato, seasonings and 2 tablespoons water. Simmer until vegetables are just tender. Sprinkly crisp bacon on top and serve.

Luncheon Salad (For 3)

1 Head Romaine
1 Stalk Celery, sliced
2 Chopped Tomatoes
4-5 Sliced green olives

1 Hard-cooked egg, grated
2/3 C Cottage cheese,
    softened with
3-4 T Skim milk

2 T Sliced green onion
2/3 C Leftover meat, fowl
   or fish, finely sliced

½ T Basil leaves
1/8 t Dried basil

Tear greens into bite-sized pieces. Combine all other ingredients. Sprinkle with basil and serve with cottage cheese as dressing.

DESSERTS

Mocha Sweets

½ Square unsweetened baking
   chocolate, grated
1 t Freeze-dried coffee
2/3 C Non-fat dry milk

1 T Dry sugar substitute
2/3 t Vanilla
2½ T Skim milk

Stir dry ingredients together. Sprinkle with vanilla and milk and stir. Shape mixture with hands into small globes or drop by teaspoon onto wax paper. Place in freezer for about 3/4 hour. Then serve.

Pudding Whip (For 1)

3 T Non-fat dry milk
2 t Lime juice
3 T Water
1 t Gelatin

Dash of cardamon
2/3 t Saccharin or sucaryl
   to taste
1½ t vanilla

Prepare gelatin by adding to water for several minutes, then dissolve over hot water. In electric mixer, beat together all other ingredients for about 15 minutes. Add gelatin mixture gradually, beating, until it forms peaks. Chill and serve.

Coffee Bavarian (4-6 Servings)

1 T Gelatin
2 C Black coffee
Sugar substitute to taste

1 t Non-fat dry milk
½ t Vanilla

Soften gelatin in cold water. Dissolve in hot coffee and add sugar substitute and vanilla. Mix well and chill until jelled. Put into blender, adding dry milk on high speed for a few seconds. Refrigerate.

Chiffon au Chocolat (5-6 Servings)

1 T Gelatin
½ C Skim milk
3 Eggs
¼ C Unsweetened cocoa

1 t Instant coffee
4 t Artificial sweetener
1 t Vanilla
¼ t Cream of tartar

Soften gelatin over ½ cup milk in pan. Beat egg yolks and milk with fork and add to pan. Mix in cocoa and coffee. Stir constantly over low heat until slightly thickens. Remove from heat and add sweetener and vanilla. Chill. Meanwhile, beat egg white with cream of tartar until it forms peaks. Fold into chilled gelatin. Place in mold. Chill several hours.

Blender Pudding (For 1)

Use any fresh fruit such as: blackberries, strawberries, gooseberries, honeydew, casaba, peach, pear, plum. Cut up enough for one portion. Sweeten to taste (non-caloric). Add 1 heaping tablespoon home-made cottage cheese (recipe follows). Blend all together until smooth and chill in serving bowl.

Strawberry Mousse (For 3-4)

2 t Gelatin	2 t Vanilla
2 T Cold skim milk	1 C Home-made cottage cheese
1 T Liquid sweetener	12 Fresh strawberries, sliced

Soften gelatin over ½ cup milk in pan. Beat egg yolks and milk with fork and add to pan. Mix in cocoa and coffee. Stir constantly over low heat until slightly thickens. Remove from heat and add sweetener and vanilla. Chill. Meanwhile, beat egg white with cream of tartar until it forms peaks. Fold into chilled gelatin. Place in mold. Chill several hours.

Home-Made Cottage Cheese

(Approximately 2 Cups)

Bring to lukewarm temperature (test on inner wrist) ½ gallon skim milk. Stir in 4 tablespoons buttermilk. Cover with linen towel and let stand in protected spot for 24 hours. Next day, line a colander with the towel and place in kitchen sink. Strain the thickened milk through the colander and let sit about 10 minutes to drain. Then set colander over a deep pot, cover with ends of the towel or plastic wrap and place in refrigerator for 24 hours more, pouring off the liquid that accumulates below from time to time. Scrape out with rubber spatula into covered dish and keep refrigerated. This creamy cheese can be used over fruits. Sweetened and with flavoring added, such as vanilla, almond or maple, it can be used as topping for desserts.

PARTY FARE

Near East Dip

1½ C Yogurt (plain)   1½ t Onion, minced
Dash of salt (or kelp),   ½ t Caraway seeds
  cumin

Blend together and chill. Serve with sliced cucumbers, raw string beans, sliced turnips, etc.

Dip a la Russe

1 Small container cottage   Small jar Caviar
  cheese   1/8 t Horseradish
¼ C Skim milk

Blend milk and cottage cheese until consistency of sour cream. Stir in the caviar and horseradish. Serve on raw vegetable slices.

The Meat of Chapter 3

Learn to spot carbohydrates and fats a mile away. Give them a wide berth before they give you a wide girth.

Learn to live in the world of nutritious proteins such as meat, poultry, fish, seafood, eggs and lower fat cheeses.

Shop, cook and eat with *you* in mind. Don't feed your guilt, shame, and self-contempt by breaking a rigid diet or exposing yourself to sweets and starches.

Eat for enjoyment and nutrition. Learn new ways to prepare meat, fish and other proteins, new ways to prepare non-thickened soups, fresh salads, leafy vegetables and tasty desserts.

I want you to enjoy eating, not suffer dieting. I'll even help you set the table.

4

THE ONE "FOOD" IN THIS PROGRAM
THAT INSURES SUCCESS

Appetizer for Chapter 4

Some people see the good in the most dismal happenings.

Some people see trouble in the most fortuitous events.

Where do you stand in the happiness spectrum?

Do you desire to increase your happiness level? In this chapter, I show you how to begin.

It will be as though you are wearing a special pair of rose-colored glasses.

And I'm not even an optometrist.

She had been married one month. Her wedding dress managed to cover her 198 pounds easily as she lost weight soon after meeting him. But after the wedding, the weight loss stopped and she was in my office—22, 5'7", and eyes of blue.

"I've been around heavy people all my life, doctor. I am used to being fat myself. But now I don't want to be overweight. My husband's family and friends are thin. He says I should do whatever pleases me. But I can see his reaction when I eat rich foods."

"What is *your* reaction when you eat rich foods?"

"I live for the moment. Then I'm sorry later. I love food, I guess."

"Do you love yourself?" I hit her in the very first minute of the first interview with a question we usually don't get around to for weeks.

"I don't want to be overweight. I hate myself for failing to lose weight. The more I try, the more I fail, and the more I hate myself."

Slender people usually don't hate themselves. Perhaps they don't love themselves as much as they should. But self-hate is one of the greatest appetite stimulants.

You can't hate yourself while you are eating. Food relieves the pain of self-hate. So why stop eating?

When you stop eating and realize what you have done, you hate yourself much more.

The pain of self-recrimination can become unbearable. How about a slice of layer cake with vanilla ice cream to forget your troubles?

So it goes. The wheel of fortune cookies.

What happens when an overweight person decides to understand, appreciate, and even love himself?

You guessed it. He begins to lose weight.

FOOD FOR THOUGHT CAN FATTEN YOU, TOO

"Doctor, I've cleaned out my refrigerator. All the wrong foods are out of my kitchen. Nothing is in my house that is not proper food for the program."

"But what is in your mind?"

It's a wonder I have any patients. I really sock it to them. But somehow they understand I am actually showing genuine concern for them. I don't enjoy seeing people suffer. That is why I am a doctor. I would rather embarrass them momentarily with a question about their innermost private thoughts than have them sweat out years of emotional struggle, physical effort, only to die before their time.

Self-hate and self-recrimination practiced daily are more fattening than a piece of pie per day. The reason is they will probably drive you to two or three pieces of pie per day, if you permit.

If you blame yourself and condemn yourself, you are setting yourself up for another go around.

"Doctor, I am so ashamed." He had regained the lost weight within six months.

"You're playing the shame-shame game," I explained. "It's fattening."

An unemployed man explains, "I turn to food as a safety valve—to let off pent up steam. It blocks my feelings of failure and numbs me for awhile. I feel degraded for not being constructive and productive."

"How about taking a hammer and saw and making some improvements around the house?"

"Yeah, Doc, I guess the exercise will burn off some calories."

He missed my point. But I jabbed him again: "Make your own job until another one comes along. Home improvements are a good investment. It's not the energy that is going to knock the weight off. You can't possibly work as hard or as fast as you are eating. But as you develop pride in your accomplishment, you will feel more satisfied with yourself and you'll eat less."

At a recent seminar on the psychological aspects of overeating held at UCLA, it was recommended that people wait a minute or more before picking up spoon or fork. This helps to build self-confidence and self-esteem. It helps the overeater to know that he can be in control. Gradually, this control can be built from one minute to several, perhaps to hours.

It is very important *you* know that you are in control. If you say you are not in control, you invite failure. If you say you are in control, you are hanging in there.

"But, Doctor, I see *me*. I see myself resolve to try, then go and blow it at the first sight of a candy bar." I hear this, or equivalent, everyday.

"You didn't blow it," I reply. "You acted on a different set of mental priorities. If you understand these priorities, you can work out a way to reshuffle them. Meanwhile, you understand yourself and accept yourself."

A person with a poor opinion of himself usually tries to build himself into a bigger person by overeating and eating enlarging foods—fats and carbohydrates.

A person with self-confidence and self-esteem is attracted to non-fattening foods.

There is no valid reason for anyone to have a poor opinion of himself.

Let me tell you a little more about this matter of self-image.

Before you finish this chapter, you will learn to love yourself—or else.

AS YOU THINK, YOU ARE

The mind can play strange tricks on the body.

The subconscious mind controls the body, heart, lungs and helps digest the food.

By reprograming the mind one can achieve dramatic improvements in such physical problems as asthma, heart conditions, gastrointestinal disorders, colitis, diabetes, and so forth. There is virtually no area of the body that cannot be relieved of unwanted symptoms by mental reprograming . . . including excess weight.

But remember I said "unwanted symptoms." If the heart problem is some type of defense mechanism, your subconscious may want to hang on to it. In such a case reprograming may have no effect except possibly to cause a conflict which you would feel as a sense of uneasiness, possibly quite intense.

Excess weight must be an unwanted physical symptom.

- You must be unhappy with your overweight condition.
- You must be able to "see" (visualize) yourself slender.
- You must be willing to accept your new, slender life style.

Now this seems totally elementary and basic. It is. Yet despite this, many are going to find, subconsciously, that they are not ready to be thin!

You are not ready to be thin because you have an image of yourself with shortcomings.

Correct this image, and the programing for fatness is released. Programing for slenderness can then begin.

This is an over-simplification.

The self-image is just the first step. There are other emotional factors in your life which need to be examined so you can handle them.

We will be looking at these later. Meanwhile we shall take a good, long look at "self-image."

YOU AND YOUR SELF-IMAGE

Your actions, attitudes, and feelings conform to your own personal self-image. See yourself as a felon and you think like one. See yourself as an overweight person and you eat like one.

It follows that all you have to do is simply change your self-image and you can be a slender person.

True. But not simple or easy.

Don't place my patients or yourself in that fictional world of easy reducing. Buy this machine. Take this pill. Try this massage. Use this bath salt. Forget it. It's never that easy.

But it can still be fun and the programing becomes progressively easier. Improving your self-image takes a little doing. But it's well worth the effort.

Where does an inferior self-image start? It is usually at an early age through parents, teachers, or friends.

A second grader who makes a "D" in reading and an "F" in arithmetic begins to see himself as a poor student. He then behaves like a poor student. Every bad grade he receives bears him out and proves he is right in thinking himself a poor student. He actually *is* a poor student.

Several years ago a number of these poor students from elementary schools in disadvantaged urban areas were placed in a special experimental class at Harvard University. They were told they were in Harvard because they were special high calibre students. From that moment on they became good students. Their classroom work at Harvard shone compared to back home. Their self-image had been abruptly changed.

So it goes. The person who feels unliked acts in a negative way that discourages acceptance. The salesman with an attitude of failure invites rejection. The positive and enthusiastic salesman inspires confidence and acceptance by his customers.

You act like the person you believe yourself to be. Your appetite "hell" is no exception.

How do you go about changing your self-image?

If I told you, you could not do it.

You heard me.

If I tell you to be happy with yourself, can you be?

If I tell you to accept yourself, can you do it?

If I tell you to hold yourself in wholesome self-esteem, is it possible for you to just go ahead and do it?

If I tell you, you cannot do it.

However, if you tell yourself how to change your self-image, you *can* do it.

If you tell yourself to be happy, it carries some weight. You respond. It carries the weight right off you.

The more convincing you are when you tell yourself you have reasons to be happy, the more you change your self-image. You do it by a process you will hear more about as we move along. It is called programing.

Two people can experience the same conditions. One can find these conditions are happy ones. The other can find the same conditions make him unhappy.

It's the old story: you can see the glass as half empty or half full.

Suppose I were to meet you on the street today and greet you with a cheery, "How are you?" What would you reply?

"Not so good, Doctor. My back has been bothering me. Maybe it's my kidneys. . . ." And on and on.

Would you give me an organ recital? Or would you echo a sunny hello?

People who walk stoop-shouldered because they feel droopy are reinforcing that droopy feeling. Were they to decide to adopt a more vital "front," the "front" would soon become the real thing.

Act happy and you change the unhappy habit.

If you change the unhappy habit, you are creating the foundation for a better self-image.

If you build a better self-image, you change your eating patterns.

If you change your eating habits, you become a new, more slender person.

Be happy. You may just start a "for want of a nail" story in reverse.

HOW TO: ACCENTUATE HAPPINESS BY DWELLING ON ASSETS RATHER THAN LIABILITIES

If you are unhappy, you are not happy. Whenever you are unhappy any moment during the rest of today, ask yourself the reason. Then check out the reason. Is it a valid reason to be unhappy? Can you think of a more valid reason to be happy at that moment; two, three, four? (The money you have instead of the money you do not have. The friends you have instead of the friends you do not have. Comforts, assets, health, beauty, job, etc.)

You will be making a beginning in this process of thinking about *you*.

Want to know something? It's going to change your life.

A.M., 46, felt sorry for herself. She had good reason. Her husband was an alcoholic and gradually killing himself. She felt he was killing her, too. She looked it. Her hair was falling out. She was always tired or sick. And she was constantly crying.

In a way it was beneficial that she gained weight, or she could have gone the way of all flesh. At 164, she decided to go on a diet because everyone else was doing it. She made the mistake of coming to me. No diet—instead, a program.

Sure, she lost weight—20 pounds in seven weeks—but what she gained far outweighed her weight loss: She began wearing a wig and manicuring her nails. She went to school to learn speech therapy. She accepted her husband's condition as an illness rather than a reaction to her—stopped crying and began smiling.

You have more to gain from this program than you have to lose.

When a woman becomes a widow at 62, it's a great crisis. She is at the crossroads of creating a new life or making the best of what's left of the old. V.C. chose the new life. But her tears kept getting in the way.

She began to lose weight on our program, but couldn't talk without crying. She would ask a question then break into tears. For several months she was a familiar sight to the other patients—red-eyed, grieving, sobbing. Fortunately, the tears did not interfere with thinking differently about herself and writing about her intentions to break into a new life.

She programed herself by dwelling on assets and viewing the bright side of life. This restored her self-confidence, self-esteem and zest for living.

Then came the breakthrough—the realization of a miracle. We saw it in the no-tears, the faint smile, the new hair-do and make-up, the youthful clothes, and the sound of a voice with hope and enthusiasm in it. She dropped 27 pounds in six months. And she gained a new life.

When a patient can't look the doctor straight in the eyes, it is often a sign that the patient cannot look at himself squarely either. I notice that patients who think about themselves and study their own eating patterns gradually begin to look you in the eye. It's a sure sign to me that they are more self-understanding and self-confident.

G.W. was cross-eyed. She was also about 40 pounds overweight. She had two reasons to avert your eyes, and avert she did. She looked down, therefore always appeared depressed and withdrawn. Within eight months she had won her own self-respect to the point the excess weight had fully melted away and she was wearing eye make-up to accentuate her direct look.

YOU CAN SELECT HAPPINESS OR UNHAPPINESS–THE CHOICE IS YOURS

When she awakened one morning, Ruth wrote:

"I am going to 'start over.' I've been down too long. I haven't been willing to do for myself whatever was necessary.

"I was not coping with frustration, disappointment, loneliness and rejection in a healthy way. I was letting it 'eat' me up. For every ounce of pain inside me, I would try and cover it with fat.

"Unrealistic and disappointing love affairs had led me to take the opposite approach–make myself unappealing by allowing myself to become fat again. It's a beautiful defense mechanism, yet ugly as hell.

"I am determined to learn to cope with my environment and to live life to the fullest. I am determined to 'make it.' I am determined to sacrifice my rut as comfortable as it may be for what I really want–happiness!

"I will drink at least eight glasses of water daily; eat protein until I shed twenty-five pounds; eat proper amounts; and exercise daily to achieve my goal by December 1st. I will obtain my goal. In my mind I know I can because I can imagine the successful results."

Can anyone miss with such feeling, enthusiasm, goal imagining and expectation of success? Ruth lost weight week after week and soon reached her slender goal.

If you dwell for a few minutes a day on the valid reasons in your life for you to be happy, you can actually create a habit of happiness.

Every morning when you awaken, there are two paths you can follow.

One path is the path of seeing the dark side of everything–the negative, the problems, the liabilities.

The other path is the path of seeing the sunny side of everything–the positive, the solutions, the assets.

Program yourself now to follow the happiness path.

HOW TO: START EACH DAY OFF ON A
POSITIVE, HAPPY NOTE

Set the book aside at the end of this paragraph and visualize yourself in bed. You are awakening. It is morning. See yourself thinking immediately about the joy of a new day. Pick a specific thing to be happy about. Feel the warm elation come over you. Do it now.

This happy feeling is more important than you may realize.

A simple change of attitude, such as seeing the good instead of the bad, can permit you to feel happiness instead of unhappiness. Also, it allows your heart to function better. And your liver. And your gallbladder. And your stomach.

In fact, psychosomatic medicine has proved that all your vital organs function better when you are happy. Better gland operation. More normal metabolism.

Would you believe a normally functioning hunger mechanism?

Are you beginning to understand?

FIVE THINKING STEPS YOU MUST TAKE NOW

If you are getting the message . . .

If you are tired of on and off dieting . . .

If you are willing to think, instead of diet, to attain permanent, slender attractiveness . . .

Then I will ask you to perform five thinking steps now.

Here are five "true" or "false" statements. Read each one. Then decide. Is it true? Or is it false? Then record your answer on a separate piece of paper:

TRUE or FALSE

#1 My overweight is an abnormality.

#2 To correct it, I must understand the cause.

#3 The cause is a hang-up, quirk, or problem that inter-
  feres with my happiness.

#4 If I think about myself and observe myself I can
  identify the cause.

#5 Once identified, the cause can be understood and
  changed.

If you have answered "true" to all five statements, you are ready to have the fat melt away.

If you have answered "false" to any one of these statements, you are not ready to proceed. Let me explain why.

#1. If you think your overweight condition is normal, you are not motivated to change it. Oh, granted you will accept a slender profile if I hand it to you on a silver platter. But, we both know it doesn't come about that way.

#2. If you think you can alter a condition without altering the cause, take another look to see what makes the world go round.

#3. Whatever interferes with happiness, interferes with the normal functioning of the body. The least you can say is "possibly true." I will accept that. Then you can eliminate the unhappiness excuse and watch your measurements shrink.

#4. If you think you cannot be your own amateur psychiatrist, then you will try to prove you can't. Say "true" and prove that answer correct.

#5. If you haven't identified the reason yet, how can you say you can't cope with it? I will accept "possbily true" here also. But I have ten dollars to your one that you are not a creature of circumstances—instead, you are a creator of circumstances.

Have you thought through these five steps?

Are you ready to endorse them as "true" or at least "possibly true?"

Those of you who haven't, stay here a while and think about it.

The remainder of you follow me.

PSYCHOLOGICAL PROFILE OF AN OVERWEIGHT PERSON

Take a look at the man over there. This is his third trip to the buffet. His plate is piled so high, he may lose part of his "treasure" before he reaches the table. No wonder he comes to an eat-all-you-want buffet—he would go broke otherwise.

Here is factual evidence that this man has a hang-up, quirk or problem. (As agreed in #3 above.)

What might it be?

I have talked with many psychiatrists, psychologists, marriage counselors, business consultants, and family physicians. In addition, I have talked with thousands of patients like our buffet-com-miting friend.

Here, in aproximate order of their frequency, are the problems, quirks and hang-ups that "bug" people in general and fat people in particular.

COMMON PROBLEMS, QUIRKS, HANG-UPS

Financial insecurity (long range)	Sexual fear
	Self-pity
Loneliness	Sexual confusion
Business pressure	Uncertainty or
Marital incompatability	indecision
Sexual frustration or difficulty	Lack of independence
Critical money problem	Hyper-activity
Boredom	Lack of adjustment to life
Self-centeredness	Hyper-sensitivity
General cynicism	Inhibitions
Despondency	Phobia about health,
Hunger for recognition	fear of death
Feelings of inadequacy	Lack of creative
Apathy	interest
Laziness	Family problem
Responsibilities	Nature of work
Guilt	Difficulty getting
Embarrassment	along with people
Nervous tension	Marital infidelity
or fatigue	Religious doubts
Conflicts in home	or indecision
or environment	Rebellion against
Other people's	society or convention
opinions	Fear of danger

This list is barely a start. Yet one or two must certainly sound familiar to you. Not that they are the direct cause of your eating abnormality. But they come close.

Develop a feeling for the general type of problem you are looking for.

What happens when you identify it?

Don't fret. It doesn't have to be taken away from you.

You will learn how to insulate the problem from your false appetite circuits—so it won't ring like a Pavlov bell.

Many people don't want to lose their problem. Their mind has dwelt on it continuously for such a long time that it is almost the same as losing a close friend.

Family vendettas go on for years. No one wants to lay the

cudgel down to forgive and forget. The seething seems to be too much fun for them.

Business men or women who finally strike it rich often try to upset the success formula. Seems as though they have a financial "death wish."

Individuals with special problems enjoy feeling sorry for themselves. They derive attention—from themselves and the refrigerator, if from nothing else.

I don't want you to feel threatened by the loss of your problem. You will be able to keep it if you wish.

The point is you cannot have your cake and eat it, too. Keep the problem. But be prepared to separate it from food.

PROBLEMS CAN MELT AWAY WITH THOSE EXCESS POUNDS

When Terry came to see me in May, she weighed 222 pounds. At 5'5", this made her about as broad as she was tall. By December she was down to 155. Then there was a change in her life:

> "When I first began this program, I had been dating a young man for several months. He seemed very anxious for me to follow the plan. He also was, and still is obese (about 150 excess pounds). As the program progressed, and I became slimmer, his attitude slowly changed. From a warm, close relationship, he became more distant and less affectionate, etc. We were often together, yet hundreds of miles apart.
>
> "He would become 'uptight' with me when he would prepare a fantastic dessert I could not eat or whenever I refused to go out for pizza with him. Soon our relationship dissolved—seeing each other less and less often, to the point of nothing.
>
> "I personally feel this is in direct response and proportion to the weight I have lost. He was being 'put on the spot' by mutual friends to 'take a lesson' from me. He knew he should do something about his own weight but was not willing. Yet, he could not tolerate the fact of my declining poundage.
>
> "I went to a seminar this weekend. During the second day I made a happy discovery. While walking down the street to do some shopping during lunch break, I found myself actually looking at my reflection in the glass windows of the stores. For years I have ardently refused to look in a mirror—I have, instead, turned my head away.
>
> "Now I am not ashamed."

Is Terry going to have more problems? Or less problems? The last time I saw her she was even slimmer and engaged to a handsome, young junior executive.

Your state of consciousness is the most important element of your life. It controls your body. It controls your personality. It attracts people, events, and circumstances.

Since you control your consciousness, your life can be a bowl of cherries (maintenance program and then only once a day).

A taxi driver gestures at you because you cut into his lane.

The boss has you retype a letter.

An important customer switches his account to your competitor.

Is it a blow to your self-esteem? Do you have an unhappiness reaction? Do you feel grumpy, irritable, resentful for hours, perhaps for days?

Your reply may be, "Doesn't everybody?"

An unhappiness reaction to untoward events is not the only course you have.

Your reaction can be to shrug it off.

"C'est la vie."

"Que sera, sera."

"You lose some, you win some."

There's a happiness reaction for unwelcome events in every language.

Unhappiness. Happiness. The choice is yours.

If you are overweight, it is probably because you are in the habit of making an unhappiness choice. So you compensate by making yourself mouth or belly happy.

This habit factor requires some perseverance to change. The choice is yours. But if you choose happiness, you may not be able to have happiness immediately—until you change the unhappiness habit.

I will be giving you some mental reprograming techniques—as easy as relaxing in a comfortable chair—to change the unhappiness habit. Then, watch problems melt away and excess pounds with them.

But, first we need to continue with our search for problems, quirks or hang-ups.

WHAT FAT PEOPLE ARE SAYING THESE DAYS

Let's listen to Mr. B.D. report about the reason for his 304 pounds:

"I need to let off steam, emotional steam. I turn to food like a safety valve. It stops my thoughts from running rampant, numbs them for awhile. Like right now I'm unemployed. It makes me feel sorry for myself. I don't think much of myself lying around the house not being productive. So I abuse myself with self-criticism, then find excuses. What I need is constructive channels for this thought energy. When I'm engaged in a satisfying job, I have no craving to run to food. Now, the moment I awaken each morning I feel defeated. Here we are with a new baby to feed and me without a job."

I ask you—when Mr. B.D. left my office after these revealing thoughts about himself, did he head for the nearby luncheonette or employment office? I don't know, but I would assume more of his energy went into thinking and job hunting.

On the other hand, here is Miss T.Z. talking to me about herself:

"I am not very proud of myself. How much did I gain—six pounds? I ran out of medicine. Also, I retain fluid before my period. If I stay away from my mother's house I do fine. I don't keep sweets or fatty things in my house. I just don't buy them. But mother keeps a lot of fatty things and insists on cooking things she knows I enjoy, like potatoes fried in corn oil. Then I just get weak. I say to myself, well, it won't hurt just this one time. I'd be better off if I stayed home. I'll just have to put my mind to it ... as of now ... must remember ... have to lose weight ... I'm determined ... I'm going to ... I want ... etc, etc."

Get the picture of T.Z? As you can imagine I could not remain silent listening to her discourse. Here are a few of my interruptions:

Can you think of any other excuses?
Will you stay home all your life?
Will you stay away from food always?
You don't keep sweets, but do you keep (take care of) yourself?

Does corn oil and French fries send out waves which overpower you?
Remember not to forget, remember to remember.
How can you put your mind to it, with glue or stickum paste?
What will you do to help yourself succeed?
Will you accept my hand if I offer to pull you out of the rut? My "hand"
    is the reading matter I gave you, the writing matter for which I have
    asked, and the program I have outlined.

Well, it wasn't easy with Miss T.Z. She attended a review lecture for extra re-programing. She began to write. It was like pulling teeth but she eventually lost more than the weight of a few elephant tusks.

Here is Mrs. S.L. talking to me through her tears:

> "I've just got to begin again. I don't want to make excuses. I don't want to go backward. It's really hard for me to come here and feel disappointed in myself. I want to succeed. I don't want to be a failure. I don't want to use you, doctor, as a crutch. I want to be strong myself. I keep putting myself on the mental hot seat. All I come up with is—I don't love myself. I don't understand myself. I don't have any mental strength."

Intersperse about every three words with a sob and you will begin to understand Mrs. S.L. I could see her playing the "back and forth" game or "on again, off again" game. What she was actually telling me between the sobs and even with the sobs was, "I feel so good when my belly is full, nothing else matters."

Did I berate her? Did I tell her she's a weakling? Did I exhort her to try harder? Did I cut her food intake? No, no, no.

I was understanding, kind and compassionate. I encouraged her to feel and think about herself the same as I did. The problem can be solved. Sweets and starches are the enemy. If you can't defeat them by direct confrontation, how about outflanking them? Get around them by thinking, thinking, thinking about yourself. Thinking at the moment you eat wrong foods, eat too much, or eat too frequently. And then writing, writing, writing.

S.L. is not crying any more. She has lost 45 pounds.

> Sometimes the benefits from losing weight are more than you realize. C.E.'s weight shrank from a whopping 238 pounds to 159 in one year on the think-about-yourself, write-about-yourself program. Later she was in a serious auto accident and suffered severe injury to her neck and back which required extensive surgery. Her orthopedic specialist told her that if she had not lost the weight, he could not have performed the surgery.

Sometimes weight changes can be dramatic, but ten pounds off fast or slow is still ten pounds off. G.M. was 20 years old, six feet tall, and wanted to enlist in the Air Force. There was one obstacle. He weighed 358 pounds. He had problems at home. His parents were divorced. Now his mother had remarried and discovered her husband was unfaithful. Well, G.M. learned how to disconnect his appetite from all this and become more independent. Results: in four months he had lost 70 pounds. The Air Force doctors couldn't believe how he had changed in body, looks, and bearing.

HOW TO RECKON WITH THE REAL CAUSE OF OVEREATING

Thinking always turns up the same discovery: food is not the basic problem. There is something else at the root of overeating. Identify the basic problem and you can eliminate the overeating by simple reconditioning.

If Pavlov's dogs were becoming fat and he stopped to analyze why, he would find that every time the clock struck the hour, the dogs would salivate. Mistaking their salivation for hunger, the dogs would hit their chow troughs. Result—too much food.

Now what could Pavlov do about it? He would have to devise a way to undo the bell conditioning he had originally created by ringing a bell when the food was placed in the troughs. Perhaps, now he would keep food in the troughs all the time and remove it just before he rang a bell and before the clock struck. Soon the dogs would no longer feel the flow of saliva at the bell or on the hour.

We have to perform some similar reprograming on ourselves once we identify our Pavlov bells. It is easy and it's fun.

It beats hunger, tears, and failure.

The person who loses a few pounds, then gives up time and time again, is creating a habit pattern. Failure reinforces failure.

Success reinforces success.

You cannot have success by tackling only the food addictions, the false hungers, and the chronic cravings. You can have success by tackling the basic causes of your eating abnormalities.

Why undertake dieting when you know ahead of time you are certain to fail, and in the process of failing, reinforce the very abnormalities you are working to eliminate?

It is easier to observe yourself—to think, analyze, consider—then abstain, not from food, but from certain thoughts or attitudes.

It is impossible to abstain from eating as you do unless you abstain from thinking or feeling as you do.

I cannot help you go successfully from 2,000 calories a day to 500 calories.

I can help you change from 2,000 unhappy thoughts a day to practically none.

It pains you to live on 500 calories a day as you well know.

It pleasures you to live on no unhappy thoughts a day, as you will find out.

And you will lose weight easily and permanently.

The Meat of Chapter 4

Identify whatever drains your cup of happiness. Inventory a number of sources of happiness. Tap these sources by thinking of them any time you observe yourself feeling sorrow or developing unhappy thoughts.

Begin the day with a happy thought. When you first open your eyes, or when you first place your feet on the floor, stop to enjoy the warm feeling that comes from picturing the good you have in life.

Admit to your over-eating and overweight being an abnormality. Resolve to identify the cause. Check off one or two common problems which strike close to home for you.

Do they ring a Pavlov bell?

When you change your attitude about such problems, you cut their connection with your appetite bell.

Break out the wire cutters.

5

HOW TO "WIRE" YOURSELF TO HEAR THE "SOUND" OF YOUR APPETITE

Appetizer for Chapter 5

Prepare for an exciting adventure. You are about to go on a mental safari.

Learn to recognize the signs that lead you to your quarry—the false appetite. Ready the weapons—thinking and writing.

Mindless eating? Its days are numbered. Prepare for the much more meaningful experience of mind-body eating.

"I use eating as a method of escape. If there's any unpleasant task I want to avoid, I look for an excuse to eat as a way of procrastinating. I've caught myself saying—first, I'll have some lunch, or—I'm thirsty—or, I need a cup of coffee (and maybe a doughnut with it). Now that I'm aware of this, I give it a second thought. Do I really need it or is it a delaying tactic?"

The words are those of L.L., a 33-year-old housewife who enjoyed a real breakthrough with this discovery about herself. After only a token loss of a pound or two a month for several months, she dropped 20 pounds in two months, ending at a svelte 125.

Mrs. L.L. found a few more "goodies" about herself by merely sitting with pen and pad and jotting down whatever came to mind:

"I resent my husband's bossing me around about my eating. I punish him. I indulge immediately in something especially fattening. . . .

"I eat out of boredom. If there's nothing special to do, Ted's not home, the children are busy, I eat as an activity. So I've taken up needlework, reading, and sculpting, and find them much more satisfying than food. . . .

"It continues to be difficult in the evening when Ted is traveling. After the children are tucked in bed, the house seems so empty. Then I move toward the cookie jar knowing this has helped. Now I move toward the salad bin and munch on celery or cucumbers with a large mug of hot coffee to keep me company."

I'm sure a lot of young housewives can see at least a part of themselves in Mrs. L.L. Every person is quite different from every other person in the reasons why they behave the way they do. But there are some common denominators.

A pound of human fat is a pound of human fat. It can come from widely different foods and even more widely different reasons for eating those foods. Put a human fat cell under the microscope and it doesn't matter whether it came from a pizza pie, a pitcher of beer or both. You will see a compound of carbon, hydrogen and oxygen. You won't see from where that compound originated—the excessive food, nor will you see the source of the excess—frustration, loneliness, insecurity, etc.

The concept that human fat springs from an excess of intake over output is valid. But we are now moving one step further: Where does this excess spring from?

Diets do work—temporarily. They cut off the excess—temporarily. End the diet and the excess returns. By definition.

But go upstream to the source of the excessive appetite and watch what happens.

HOW TO CHOKE OFF AN EXCESSIVE APPETITE
AT ITS SOURCE BY GOING ON A MENTAL SAFARI

The source of excess—be it food or drink or sex or smoking—lies in feelings, thoughts and emotions.

I take my patients on a mental safari. We track the cause of excess. Once we find it, we cage it, contain it. No more excess.

This mental safari does not require guns or ammunition. Its weapons are pen and paper.

Instead of hiking and shooting, you think and write.

Mrs. L.L.'s remarks were the result of this kind of a mental hunting trip. Hers was a successful safari.

For some I do not advise such a safari without competent guides. There can be mental country where the going is rough.

Persons with severe traumatic experiences in their background should not attempt self-analysis as it could easily open a Pandora's box of frightening memories. However, the majority of us will find a mental safari an exciting mental adventure—one leading to vital discoveries and understanding about one's self.

The more we know about ourselves, the more we are able to face life without shames, without guilts, without doubts and move forward toward the goals of happiness and affluence that we set.

E.R., a single girl aged 26, had an inate attractiveness barely visible through her 194 pounds when she came for help. After two months she had lost only 4½ pounds. No, she said, she didn't have time to think or write about herself. I gave her hell. Pulled no punches. I'll spare you the details. But in two weeks she came back with this:

"After the severe tongue lashing from you, Dr. Schiff, and after much self-observation and self-analysis, I arrived at this conclusion: my appetite goes haywire when I become aware that other people are disappointed in me or when my security is at stake. (For instance, due to my definitely knowing your disappointment with me, I couldn't leave food alone for more than a week, my hands erupted with a rash from nervousness, my face appeared as though adolescence was upon me again. I was a mess!)

"Basically, I am a highly insecure person although at times no one would know from outward appearances. But with only a slight reprimand or 'anti-me' statement, my shell can be cracked and my emotions take over. I may become highly defensive of myself or degrading of another to make myself appear without blemish.

"I have found myself doing this at work when I've made an error or when I have offended someone by my trap being open once too often. And in all sorts of situations such as finances running low, a loss of a beau, unexpected car trouble, or simply the inability to accomplish what I thought I could, my insecurity takes control.

"Then I find myself running to the refrigerator, opening mouth, and inserting food. It evidently serves as a means of escape.

"This is the first time I have thought about this. Being made to think has made me realize I want to eat when I am dissatisfied with myself, or I've placed myself in a displeasing situation which will affect my security in financial, vocational, social or personal matters. I think it has been a healthy trip."

It was the breakthrough for which I was searching. She was thinking about herself in a way that she probably never did before. It was obviously a new adventure in living for her. She also enjoyed this mental trip or safari. She slapped this typed account into my hands triumphantly as though it was a trophy of elephant tusks worth a thousand dollars.

Then her weight loss increased six or seven pounds every two weeks. She soon reached her desired weight and shifted to the maintenance program.

Now don't misunderstand. All this did not happen because of this one record of self-examination. E.R. continued to think. Any time she was tempted to eat between meals, to take an overly large portion or a second portion, or to pop a snack in her mouth, she stopped to think. Then she recorded her thoughts. This process did not stop until she went on the maintenance program.

Even then, any display of appetite, as opposed to hunger, would be the signal for another mental safari.

SIGNS THAT LEAD YOU TO THE QUARRY ON YOUR MENTAL SAFARI

If you were to set this book aside in order to write all about yourself and why you eat the way you do, you would probably stare at the paper for some time. It's similar to recalling a dream in the afternoon. It is much easier to recall and write about a dream in the morning when you awaken, closer to the time it happens.

Similarly, it's easier to recollect and write about the urge to gorge beyond the call of duty as you are experiencing that urge.

Here is a list of "danger" times—times when the bars may go down and nibbling, overeating, or faulty eating may occur.

Read the list. Mark the times that appear to fit into your lifestyle. Then resolve that you will *write*, not eat, if that moment arrives:

- Cooking or working in the kitchen.
- Cleaning after a meal and storing leftovers.
- Opening the refrigerator.
- Being with others who are snacking.
- Buying fattening foods in the supermarket.
- Storing foods after shopping.
- Visiting relatives or friends.
- Eating in restaurants.
- Attending parties or social functions.
- On the go and too rushed to eat properly.
- Having a coffee or snack break.
- Entertaining at home.
- Arriving home from work or school.
- Watching TV, listening to the radio, hi-fi.
- Being alone at night or anytime.
- Doing housework, homework or any type of work.
- Writing letters, sewing, reading.
- Talking on the telephone or with friends.
- Bored with nothing to do.
- Seeking a reward or pick-me-up after a hard day.
- Coping with a crisis, coping with yourself.
- Worrying about a problem, being "bugged" by something or someone.
- Finding that the scale shows no weight loss after you behaved so well.

Are you bored now? Is your mind turning to something to eat—something more toothsome than celery or carrot sticks? Good. Reach for pen and paper instead and describe the feeling.

Remember those cigarette ads? "Reach for a _____ instead of a sweet." This may be as if you jumped out of the frying pan into the fire.

But you cannot go wrong reaching for a pen instead of a pizza—and writing instead of eating. You are opening doors to a a slimmer self.

You're tired. You decide a cup of coffee is just what the doctor ordered. You are fine so far. Then, waiting for the water to boil, you remember that box of cookies. Hold it. That's not what the doctor ordered.

Why must something go with the coffee? Think back. Reason it. Develop insight and understanding. Then write about it.

It could sound similar to this:

"I've been good. I've worked hard. ('Mommy, can I have a cookie?' 'Sure, darling, you've been such a good child. Take some milk with it.') I'm happy with myself—such a good worker. I'll have a couple of cookies with the coffee."

However it comes out, writing about it requires thinking and understanding what it is all about. Thinking about it changes it.

How does thinking about it change it? Well, what you are really doing is dragging it out of the dark recesses of the subconscious mind into the hot, white light of your critical scrutiny.

Connecting the cookie to a childhood reward by thinking about it is really saying, "Isn't that ridiculous? Why, I'm no child any more. I don't need a cookie for a reward."

This conscious, critical analysis takes cookie programing out of the activating portion of your subconscious mind. For years this has been making you behave in a way that leads to excessive weight. Instead, you are refiling it in the subconscious mind under an inactive, non-behaving file heading, we might call "obsolete."

Result: The next time you feel like having a cup of coffee and the cookie idea crops up, you are likely to get a few chuckles out of it instead of a few fat cells.

The benefits are endless.

Here's how one woman describes the extra health benefits she enjoyed after dropping only a few pounds. "When I changed my thinking, things began to happen to me. I was able to discontinue the medication for high-blood pressure as it dropped. I have more pep and energy. My leg cramps have disappeared and my varicose veins have improved. I'm not the nervous person I used to be."

Writing and thinking about herself allowed this patient to gain access to her subconscious mind. Her new found awareness helped achieve the miracles described above.

Sometimes, beneath the layers of fat, lie undiscovered talents.

You couldn't see C.S. at work. You could only talk to her—she was a service representative for the telephone company. Just as well. She had a bad complexion and poor teeth. Nice features disappeared in her pudgy face.

In five months her weight only went from 133 to 123, but C.S. was a different person. Her complexion cleared; her fingernails grew and didn't break; her teeth were capped; and her face was angelic. She became interested in many things. She found she had a great talent in art. She left the phone company and became a successful free-lance artist.

Ten or twenty pounds can make a difference in a woman's appearance. But the miracle is the new way she sees herself. Her self-image can change from one of hopelessness to one of hope. With H.B., a 29-year old divorcee, 18 pounds off her weight was great, but long before the scales showed this, her own opinion of herself had changed. This was evidenced by:

- Mod clothes
- Contact lenses
- Several wigs
- New job

Just another word about picking the time to think and write. Often the time picks you, as it did for Mrs. L.J.:

"Many overweight people such as me try to brainwash themselves into thinking they are not actually *too* fat. My day of awareness came with a completely innocent reaction by my husband. It was a Saturday morning, my husband had the day off from work. I had just stepped out of the bathtub. I decided I would alluringly entice my husband, who was still in bed, by walking in with only a pair of polka-dot bikini panties.

"As I entered the bedroom, wearing my most fetching smile, my husband looked up from his morning newspaper and began to laugh hysterically. He couldn't stop for about five, long, agonizing minutes.

"That did it. I decided then and there to take the safety pin out of my mind and put it in my skirt."

Of course, Mrs. L.J. didn't sit down to think and write while her husband was still rocking with laughter. But you can be sure it wasn't much later when she began.

MEDITATING ON YOUR WEIGHT CAN BE ENLIGHTENING

Many people prefer to pick their own time to think about themselves. That's fine, too. I mentioned the best times because the meat of the problem—or should I say the sweet of the problem?—was close at hand, the better to be observed.

You may prefer a time when the kids are off to school and the beds are made, or when you have a weekend or evening hour to yourself.

Since there may be no specific incident other than developing a line of thought—such as the cookie with the coffee—you must do some mental free wheeling. It is like starting on a mental safari without a trail to follow.

Mrs. A.A. placed a piece of paper upon the cocktail table as she sat back comfortably on the couch to think about her weight. She found herself reflecting upon her two marriages in a way she had never done before, almost like a mirror reflecting her own physical image.

Thoughts can be so fleeting they can escape and become lost forever. Mrs. A.A. remembered my advice to "write it down," to capture the thoughts on a mental safari. She began writing:

> "We were married nine years and it was a constant struggle. He was in college most of the time. At the end of nine years, we separated and soon were divorced.
>
> "My world was shattered. I was heartbroken. I gathered my children and moved in with my family back east. Though they were well situated, I went to work. Then I began eating sweets. I was very unhappy—I think the sweets helped me forget my problems. I never talked to anyone about my unhappiness and pretended to be happy.
>
> "Then I met and married another man. I didn't love him. I only married him because he could provide rather well for me and my children. I soon realized what a wonderful person he was. Now I love him more than I ever dreamed possible. But I doubt he would think much of me if I could not control my weight."

This is the written result of her first meditation on her life as it related to her weight. Did it come out right? Did she really hit around the crux of the problem?

Apparently she did. She became less compulsive about sweets and more motivated to restore her natural beauty.

> "I am beginning to think more about myself," she told me later. "I feel more important. I don't become depressed. I see myself becoming more attractive."

Meditation may be a frightening word to some people—too heavy. That's why I also use "mental safari." This term may also turn off some people—too much like living dangerously. How about using your own word for it? The important thing is to do it.

Make yourself comfortable.

Think about yourself.

Write it down.

NOW GIVE "EQUAL TIME" TO THE SOLUTION

Once you have written about your eating problem, you're ready to write the next "chapter"—the solution to your eating problem.

How do you plan to overcome a specific problem? Suppose you were Mrs. A.A. Would you attempt to establish better communication with your husband? If so, how? Would you confide in him about your efforts to lose weight and seek his support?

Write about your strategy. What reasoning will you employ to overcome your problems now that you have stalked them back to their source?

Suppose you drop over to a friend's house for coffee every Monday morning to chat about your respective weekends and plans for the week. Your friend usually insists you have a piece of pastry "from your favorite bakery" or "that I've made just for you." In the past you have accepted the starchy invitation. Your meditation notes indicate you eat these pastries despite their taboo on your program because you "do not want to hurt her feelings" and you "want to be loved."

Now, what are you going to do about it? Obviously, something must be done before next Monday.

Back to thinking. Ah, you have it. You will politely refuse the pastries while you praise the coffee for its perfect flavor and aroma. Then you will sip the coffee slowly, maybe have another cup or two, until the pastries disappear from you, back into the kitchen, or you from them.

Now pick up your pen. Record this solution on paper. Writing about it is the first step in making the solution "official" and *activating* it.

Thoughts slip away. A written record is the beginning of actualization.

You make it come alive.

YOUR MIND MADE YOU OVERWEIGHT AND
YOUR MIND CAN MAKE YOU THIN

Everything in our civilization begins with a visual thought which is then recorded on paper—a design for a new dress, a blueprint for a new boat, a sketch for a new patent. Writing it on paper captures it. Then the next step can be taken—making it come true.

In a later chapter you will learn a simple method to accelerate the *activation* of a solution. This method harnesses the powers of the mind to bring about the solution.

For instance, in the case of the Monday coffee klatch, you would "play" the scene ahead of time in your imagination. You see yourself having coffee with Helen, your friend . . . now she is bringing out the pastry platter . . . "You'll love them" . . . "You're a dear for serving them, but no thanks. Helen, this coffee is simply marvelous. You do make such delicious coffee" . . . Helen smiles graciously . . . you sip your coffee slowly . . the conversation continues. . . .

You will learn a technique to make this imagination exercise etch itself into your mind in such a manner that it can happen *only* that way. The solution you write now, and later "play" in your imagination, happens just as you imagined it. No will-power. No aimless discipline. Just easy, enjoyable *living* on your slenderizing program.

So the solution you write about can be a picture of how you now allow things to happen instead of the way they are happening. Don't be concerned now that you may be unable to act the way your solution specifies. I promise to show you a way to make it happen effortlessly.

The essential point is for you to create a picture in your solution that you can "play" in your mind as you would a movie. I promise you it will be a movie in which you star.

And it will have a happy ending.

HOW TO WRITE THE SCRIPT FOR MENTAL MOVIES
ABOUT YOURSELF WHICH BECOME STUNNINGLY REAL

Suppose you were to write on the left side of the paper how you have been eating in the past. Then, suppose you were to write on the right side of the paper how you will eat under this permanent mind-body program. Would it look something like this?

WHICH SIDE WOULD YOU
PREFER TO LIVE ON?

PROBLEM	SOLUTION
Non-diet Days	*Weight Loss Days*
Waffles and syrup	Scrambled eggs
Sandwich	Cheese blintzes
Hot dogs	Clam bisque
Pizzas	Broiled fish steak
Ice cream	Lamburger
Chocolate cake	Baked tomatoes
Diet Days	Orange sherbet
Skim milk	Spanish omelet
Can of diet mixture	Curry of cod
Carrot sticks	Braised loin of veal
Cottage cheese	Broiled lamb chops
	Maple bavarian cream
Non-diet Days	*Weight Maintenance Days*
Danish pastry	French toast
Spaghetti	Egg Louisiana
Coke	Cheese fondue
Candy bar	Spring salad
Malted	Sea food en coquille
Sandwich	Deviled salmon
Diet Days	Beef romano
Skim milk	Hungarian goulash
Can of diet mixture	Braised lamb pot roast
Carrot sticks	Chicken cacciatore
Cottage cheese	Strawberry mousse
	Ginger melon mold

Take a long look at the left side of the page. Note the cycles. Diet days. Non-diet days. Fast food. Mouth food.

You can remain on the left side of the page, if you want. It is the yo-yo syndrome. On again, off again diets as your weight goes up and down—down only after soul-searching days of "I'll start my diet tomorrow."

It is really mindless eating.

Now take a long look at the right side of the page. No cycles here. First those corrective weight (and fat) loss days. Then those permanent weight maintenance days. And what delectable eating! Perhaps less impulse food. But certainly food that is enjoyed by both your body and your mind, not just your mouth.

It is mind-body eating.

Well, which side of the page would you like to eat on? I don't want to influence your choice, but let me remind you, that while you may be occasionally slim on the left side regimen, choose the right side and you will be permanently slim.

Again, without my influencing your choice, remember that wide ups and downs in weight are a strain on vital organs; long periods of overweight take years off your life expectancy, and your whole level of well-being rises as your excess weight drops.

But I don't want to influence your decision.

H.J. was a designer but he didn't do a very good job on himself. He was a short 5'4" and a fat 227. His weakness was beer, hot dogs, taco and beans. When he came into our program, he set a goal of 130 pounds. When I last saw him he still had several pounds to lose but I'm sure he made it. H.J. dropped 71 pounds in six months. His self-examination and reprograming of his eating habits had reinforced many of his innate strengths—one of them: the strength to pass by those frank and taco stands.

When you think about yourself, yourself does not usually let you get away with fuzzy, illogical reasoning. P.H. was above her clerk job and she knew it. It depressed her. So she ate. When she thought about it, she changed her dress style, hair style and life style. She became a bookkeeper in a sportswear factory and her mind had a chance to prove what it could do. The 25 pounds she lost in the process was just incidental.

"I used to believe I calmed myself eating sweets. Now I realize I just harmed myself." D.J. calls this a turning point in the program for her. At first she didn't want to give up sweets as they were her sedative. But the more she thought and wrote about it, the more she saw sweets in their true light.

She enjoyed other benefits: less depression, had more energy, required less sleep, had a clearer complexion.

"There are good things in life when you see past personal problems. I don't need to gorge to cope with problems. I can resolve them with insight, insight I would have lost by gorging over them. I wake up each day looking forward to life's challenges."

Presumably, you are now doing something wrong about deciding what goes into your mouth. You may not be eating exactly as the left side of the page portrays. It has been exaggerated to make a point. But you are eating mindlessly. It is called mouth eating.

All you must do to arrive at the right hand side of the page is to let your mind, not your mouth, be your guide.

Are you beginning to follow the plot?

Would you like to write your own script?

It can be a stirring drama—one in which you will not be stirring cake mix batter or waffle batter, but savory sauces, fondues and stews. It will be a drama in which you emerge as a new person, and you won't need a make-up artist to turn the trick.

Here's how you write the script.

On the left side of the paper, set down the basic parts to your problem. Opposite each part write the solution to help solve the problem. It's as simple as that.

Some examples:

PROBLEM	SOLUTION
I find Saturdays rather boring. My husband golfs or works. Maybe deep inside this irritates me, too. At any rate, I eat.	I know my husband works long, hard hours for the family and needs an outlet such as golf. Maybe I'll take up golf, too, or tennis, or crocheting, or weaving.
When I cook I can't resist tasting. I simply can't wait to try different recipes. I'm stuffed by the time I sit down to eat, but I eat anyhow.	From now on tasting means just that. I will use only the tip of the teaspoon and catch the flavor the very first time. If I add an ingredient I will taste again, using only the tip of the spoon.
I go on binges for certain foods. I can have a pizza mood or chocolate mood and eat a whole pie or a whole box.	I will observe these moods, learn why they arise, and head them off before they head me off. I will also substitute proper foods for the culprit foods, preferably those on my "eat all you want" list.

Many problems you place in the script will appear to involve your family or friends and beyond your control. Don't believe this for a moment. Every problem is within your power to solve.

Researchers have found young people in upper socio-economic groups are thinner than those in lower socio-economic groups.

You, too, may have society and your environment contributing to your habits of eating more than you are contributing. Family, friends, cultures, habits, ethnic ways—all are pushing your weight up.

What do you do? Drop out?

No. You drop in. You substitute your own good sense to develop new eating habits. You insert your plan for yourself in place of society's plan.

You write the script yourself.

Meat of Chapter 5

Keep a list of danger times when extra snacking or over-eating takes place.

Write about your thoughts and feelings which seem to trigger the urge to eat. Reach for a pen instead of a pizza. You probably won't want the snack later as the triggering moment leaves. But the value of writing is much deeper than that.

Think about a solution for each danger time—a way to circumvent the particular circumstances which trap you.

Write the script for your own eating in life. Substitute it for the one society and environment has written for you.

Give me a leading part.

6

PITFALLS INTO WHICH
FAT PEOPLE FALL THE HARDEST

Appetizer for Chapter 6

The road to your weight goal is strewn with pitfalls which attract, induce and beckon. What does one do about any pitfall, be it sex, poker or shortcake? One can post warning signposts to mark them well. One can detour around them. And one can throw pitfalls in front of the pitfalls. You will see what I mean in Chapter 6.

"Marty, you'll never motivate people to think and learn about themselves by reading a book. You can help your patients. They see you face to face. You know how to encourage them. But a book. . . ?"

This was a friend whose opinion I valued. When he left the house I decided to do a little meditating myself. In fact, I decided to practice what I preach and to write about my thoughts.

Here are the results:

"I am thinking now. I am thinking about how I can help a person miles away through my writing. Especially, how I can activate his mind. How I can motivate him to think about himself as I am now thinking about myself.

"Why am I thinking about myself? Because I want and can reach a goal—sharing this easy method of permanent slenderizing with all who need it by means of a book.

"So I must motivate this person miles away to set goals as he reads. He will then have reasons to think how to reach his goal.

"My goal is this book. To help this overweight person off the treadmill of diets and on to reprograming for a Pavlov bell-free eating program. I will reach my goal. But will he (or she) set, and reach his goal?"

At this point I "free associated." Psychiatrists often ask their patients to simply talk about anything that flows through their mind. I found myself doing this:

"Beyond the light that I discovered on a hillside, I gather *me*. In the fires of my dialogue, I will find a few small flames of truth for the person I don't know. He has a weight problem. He is steeped in despair. He must discover and understand his own solar system—the mental universe he lives in.

"He has his own think tank. My think tank can fathom only me. His think tank is the only think tank that can reach the depths of him.

"But there are signposts that point the way. There are 'sharp curve ahead' signs, and 'steep grade' signs and 'slippery when wet' signs. I can provide him with many signs as he thinks along the way to enlightenment. I can help him spot pitfalls into which overweight people fall and I can help light the way with examples and case histories in order that he may better see himself.

"I can . . . I can . . . I can . . . ."

So here I am with you. Not able to think for you. Not able to give you a magic formula that points to the basic cause of your overeating. Not able to tell you specifically what to do about that basic cause or exactly how to disconnect it from your appetite.

But here I am able to tell you about:

- How others have thought and are thinking "into" themselves.
- What basic reasons they are finding.
- Successful ways they have disconnected the causes from the bell.

You can accomplish in your life the same miracles they are accomplishing in theirs.

H.H. did not enjoy his job. He was a dog catcher. At 46, he was always tired. When he came to the office in his uniform he appeared old and beaten by life. "Is that a World War I uniform?" one woman asked Linda, my nurse.

Why was H.H. gaining weight? Why was he lacking interest at home and causing his marriage to go on the rocks?

In two months, H.H. had the answer. The Pavlov dog-conditioning bells which drove him to overeat were the dogs he was chasing all day. Concurrently, with this realization, his weight dropped from 204 to 173. He found a new job as a security guard. He appeared handsome in his new uniform. His marriage was going great and from the way H.H. joked, laughed and kidded around with the nurses, I assumed he felt more alive. "You're right, Doc. It's like I'm a teenager. It's unbelieveable—almost like a miracle!"

Can children respond to this self-analysis? Or, do you have to put them in culinary handcuffs? H.L. was 11 when her mother brought her in. I can still hear her sullen "I don't care." She couldn't sit still in the office and I could readily understand why she disliked herself.

"The kids call her names and ridicule her," her mother confided.

H.L. became very interested in this business of programing new eating habits. In two months her weight went from 156 to 128. She soon wore her sister's more sophisticated clothes and became interested in swimming and bike riding.

Children have different problems and different caloric solutions to them. They often respond to introspection as readily as adults.

Senior citizens should realize it's never too late to benefit from a lighter load to carry around. G.E. was 71 when she came to the office. A tiny woman, only 4'11", she weighed 156. She continued to be active as a nursing assistant and it was taking a toll on her legs. She complained about cramps, varicose veins and arthritis. Also, her blood pressure was very high.

In five months this tired old lady had dropped 36 pounds. Her legs no longer bothered her, nor did she tire as easily. Arthritic pains disappeared and blood pressure normalized. She moved out of her daughter's apartment into one of her own. She found gentlemen friends. She not only looked and felt but also acted years younger.

PLACE YOURSELF ON MENTAL ALERT

When you turn your radio or television dials to the correct wavelength, your set begins to receive the station or channel you are seeking.

When you tune your mind similarly, you also pick up whatever you want.

If you tune your mind to ideas as to what you are next going to say to your friend, almost without any quiet time passing at all, you are able to maintain a running conversation.

If you tune your mind to a problem such as what to prepare for dinner—dinner ideas come.

Now, if you tune your mind to the question "What do I need to know about myself and my eating habits to help me normalize them?"—answers will come. Permit them to come, then . . .

Capture them. The only way to capture thoughts is to write about them immediately. If you don't write instantly, they slip away.

These are important thoughts. They are worth years of your life and tons of happiness.

You can be more specific. You can tune your mind to:

- "What pitfalls must I watch for in relation to food and eating?"
- "What triggers my appetite (false hunger)?"
- "What can I do to expose myself minimally to these appetite triggers?"

Once you develop similar mind revealing questions, you will learn the answers to some of the problems you create as the cause of an over-active appetite. I'm not saying these are your reasons but here are some that my patients have turned up:

- Sexually unresponsive mate
- Fear of meeting new people
- Inability to have orgasm
- Worry about earthquakes
- Anxiety over children leaving home

When these causes were identified by their own thinking, they were then able to tune their minds to answers as to what to do about the condition. Success in tuning their minds to pitfalls and discovering them and success in tuning their minds to causes and identifying them, reinforced their ability for success in coping with the causes.

So, in a way, you are not only normalizing your eating by thinking and writing, you are also placing yourself in a position to normalize your life.

Previously, I said you can keep your problem if you desire. I also said you can normalize your eating and your weight even though you don't eliminate the basic cause.

Now I'm saying it is possible you may hit the jackpot!

By thinking about yourself and jotting down your thoughts, you may slenderize your body and liquidate a serious problem to boot.

Largely because of his 392 pounds, R.L., 25, had many problems. One problem seemed to feed on the other and he fed on them all.

His overweight condition began with puberty some ten years ago. After high school, he opened a small auto parts shop. When he came to me, he was depressed and chronically ill with colds, insomnia, dizziness, shortness of breath, and nervousness. He said his weight was now interfering with his happiness and everyone seemed to be against him.

In the first four weeks he dropped 33 pounds. You couldn't lift the total amount of blubber he eventually gave up—150 pounds of it. It required 22 additional months until he reached 238, which looked good on his six foot frame.

They say inside every fat man is a skinny one trying to climb out. I never saw this so vividly as with R.L. He emerged confident, youthful, and energetic. His business improved. His health improved. Insomnia, dizziness and difficulty breathing also improved. And, he bragged, his social life improved.

A six feet three college basketball star added more than 60 pounds in the ten years since he graduated. At 32 and 287 pounds he was injuring his health and shortening his life. High blood pressure and a rapid pulse were the danger signs. He decided to do something about it.

He drank, ate, and smoked excessively. He was an "excessive" person. Why? He thought about it, wrote about it, read what he wrote and thought some more. The culprit: job pressures. He programed out "excess." He steeled himself to cope with pressures and transform them into challenges—like a game to be won.

Then all three excesses decreased. He smoked less than half a pack a day. He drank only socially. And in 14 weeks his weight was close to a normal 228. Naturally, his pulse and blood pressure were no longer excessive either.

LET'S GO ONE DAY AT A TIME

Today, someone once discovered, is the first day of the rest of my life.

Today is very important in our weight (and fat) loss program, and weight maintenance program.

Alcoholics Anonymous have an excellent plan for "today." If there were an Appetites Anonymous, this plan would hold just as excellently:

JUST FOR TODAY

JUST FOR TODAY I will live through this day only and not tackle my whole life problem at once. I can do something for twelve hours that might appall me if I had to keep it up for a long, long time.

JUST FOR TODAY I will be happy. Most people are as happy as they make up their minds to be.

JUST FOR TODAY I will adjust myself to what is, and not try to adjust everything to my own desires. I will take my "luck" as it comes and fit myself to it.

JUST FOR TODAY I will strengthen my mind. I will study. I will learn something useful. I will not be a mental loafer. I will read something that requires effort, thought and concentration.

JUST FOR TODAY I will do somebody a good turn, and not get found out. I will do at least two things I don't want to do—just for exercise. I will not show anyone that my feelings are hurt; they may be hurt, but today I will not show it.

JUST FOR TODAY I will be agreeable. I will look as well as I can, dress becomingly, talk low, act courteously, criticize not one bit, not find fault with anything and not try to improve or regulate anybody except myself.

JUST FOR TODAY I will have a program. I may not follow it exactly, but I will have it. I will save myself from two pests: hurry and indecision.

JUST FOR TODAY I will have a quiet half hour all by myself, and relax. During this half hour, some time, I will have a better perspective of my life.

JUST FOR TODAY I will be unafraid to enjoy what is beautiful and to believe that as I give the world, so the world will give to me.

Let me start you off on a plan for today. First I will give you a few suggestions, then you may wish to add a few of your own.

HOW TO: TEN COMMANDMENTS FOR BEGINNING A MIND-BODY PROGRAM TO SLENDERIZE ONCE AND FOR ALL

JUST FOR TODAY

- As soon as I discover myself dwelling on an unhappy matter, I will switch and dwell instead on some more joyous thought.

- I will write about my unhappy feelings and thoughts and what I switched to, developing more and more insight each time.
- I will write at every urge to eat improperly and record my thoughts and feelings at the time frankly and in depth.
- I am above feeling guilty or remorseful if I eat improperly. I understand this to be an abnormality, the cause of which I am in the process of correcting and removing.
- I will eat with others whenever possible. I have nothing to hide about my eating. It is becoming more normal every day.
- I will think more about my strengths, less about my weaknesses. I know I have nothing to fear except fear itself.
- I will eat all I need, enjoying high protein foods and developing a natural dislike for sweets, fats and starches.
- I will be constantly aware of my abilities to do helpful work and I will gain satisfaction in doing that work however humble it may be.
- I will develop more and more awareness of the real Me, the inner self that is endowed with inherent greatness of a very unique nature.
- I will accept life as it comes and make the best of it, knowing that by so doing I am creating an even better tomorrow.

Before proceeding I would ask you to do two things:

1. Read these ten commandments aloud, expressing in the tone of your voice the affirmation you feel.
2. Read these ten commandments again to yourself, stopping after each and visualizing yourself completing each one successfully.

Just for today. Just for today.

Does this have a familiar ring?

"Just this once." "Just this one time won't hurt."

When you said "just this once" and popped a chocolate in your mouth, you know where it led you.

So there is a purpose in my "just for today." If you will cooperate with yourself just for today, it will set the stage for similar cooperation tommorrow.

Cooperate on all ten points today, and you may not have to think twice about cooperating tomorrow.

Then comes a world of new tomorrows with you more slender with each successive one.

MAKE PITFALLS TURN INTO WINDFALLS

I enjoy life. I want to help others who bear the unhappy cross of obesity to lay it aside and enjoy life, too.

How can I talk about pitfalls and still be cheerful, lighthearted and joyous? Well, I think I just pulled it off.

Look back. Can you see a pitfall avoided in each of these ten commandments?

Pitfall No. 1. Dwelling on the unhappy aspect of circumstances. You have done this. You know how you dig yourself in deeper this way.

Pitfall No. 2. Turning your back on your feelings and thoughts. You know this pit. It's dark in there. No insight.

Pitfall No. 3. Eating impulsively. The first thing that comes to mind, comes to mouth.

Pitfall No. 4. Feeling guilt and remorse builds a road to that immense chasm: continued failure.

Pitfall No. 5. Secretive eating reinforces eating as an abnormality. Be willing to take your eating out of "solitary" and place it under the light of human understanding and control.

Pitfall No. 6. Fear is an ever darkening snake pit. Self-confidence and assurance banishes fear.

Pitfall No. 7. Fat is fat; the sweeter the taste, the more bitter the after-taste.

Pitfall No. 8. Laziness breeds a fat body and a fat head. You will still fit because it's a big pit.

Pitfall No. 9. Being without a philosophy concerning your spiritual identity leaves you with nothing but a body to feed.

Pitfall No. 10. By seeing the dark side of life, you build a black future.

Do you see the connection between these ten pitfalls and the ten commandments? They sound better as commandments. I asked you to re-read the commandments, but I don't want you to re-read these ten pitfalls. I wouldn't have mentioned them at all except that it is often valuable to see (visualize) the positive and negative sides to thoughts and problems.

The person who dwells on the negative aspects can become so involved in them that he never realizes there is a positive side from which to choose.

I say—choose a "yes" commandment for healthful, joyous living each time, rather than a "no" warning about dire trouble ahead.

Turn pitfalls into windfalls with that simple choice.

Exercise your franchise today. Vote "yes."

SET A ROUTE TO YOUR GOAL THAT
CIRCUMVENTS PITFALLS

Take a look inside Frances. She'll hold the flashlight for you in the form of this record of her own insight. She's 29 and, at the time of writing this, had come within ten pounds of her 130 pound goal. This had required several months and a total loss so far of about 20 pounds:

"I reach my goal of 130 and what then?

"Will people find me more interesting? Will I possess a dynamic personality? What does this final overcoat of fat hide?

"Do I resist it? That final, last, simple effort to lose eight, ten or twelve pounds. I am comfortable with my excuse—life would be happier if I were only slim. What if I found that a lean, trim shape only brought me to the realization that my weight has little to do with my problems of communication, fear, and confusion with who I am?

"Fat—I have used it to avoid relationships, to avert the closeness I have feared will bring some person so close to me that he will see my ugly soul. In my teens, with much emotional confusion, I protected myself with layers of fat. I repulsed. But I slimmed down again. For what? To be able to compete. To fit myself into the role of marriage that society expected of me because I couldn't find a role more compelling.

"I hated my role as his wife. Again, gained ten, fifteen pounds to keep Bill away. Drive him away. Repulse him. Because I could not explain that I had grown beyond him, that he was no longer a person I could love.

"At last, shedding him, sending him away. Losing twenty pounds in Europe to compete again.

"But Bill came back to marry a slim me, the one he had known at first. And then? The weight again—to prevent a struggle to remain faithful? To push him away again? I have used it to maintain the fidelity I promised, to avoid a conflict of human relations, to find a more palatable reason for failures. To excuse myself.

"I will come to grips with that turmoil. I will discover who I am. But . . . I work against myself. I watch the scale drop and run, in real fear, disguising it as some mystical need for sugar, to a bakery. Hating myself for doing it but keeping my protective layers intact."

Frances seems to have accepted something about her overeating which she discovered by meditating and writing about her thoughts in the early weeks of her program: she fattens herself to drive away her husband. Today, she writes about it easily. She also admits to fear that her "protective layers" may not be kept intact.

Suppose Frances were to go to work, would it be more difficult for her to lose weight? Until she changes her attitude toward her marriage, it will be.

The more your daily activities expose you to the problem that is driving you to food, the more you will eat.

Frances chose to keep her attitude about personal relationships. But she had to expose herself less to others in order to minimize her problems. She managed to do this through a carefully regulated social life and a carefully selected job.

If there are pitfalls which suggest excessive eating to you, why set a course right through them?

Though roots of bushes and trees have the strength to push their way through concrete and to crack rocks, they first send runners out to find a course around such obstacles.

I am going to suggest how to eliminate the impulse to eat when you are not hungry.

These impulses are triggered by programed reactions within you to outside stimuli, similar to Pavlov's bells.

These outside stimuli are simply pitfalls.

Don't rest with my warning signs. They are of necessity oriented more directly to food. Find pitfalls within yourself that relate to your hang-ups. Frances is routing her life away from exposure to men.

What must you steer clear of?

Here are some obvious eating pitfalls and how to avoid them:

- Don't skip a meal. This is a pitfall though it seems to be a most angelic act. It is this very beneficent appearance that prompts you to reward yourself. Result: two extra meals, or equal, as a reward for one meal skipped.
- Relieve boredom with fun, not food. Set a course around boredom pitfalls by making other pastimes available. A few possibilities, but not necessarily your "bag," could be a pack of playing cards or other solitaire puzzles or games strategically placed between your favorite chair and the kitchen; a list of people to whom you owe a telephone call or a letter; an interesting book; or a hobby.

- Switch your social life away from eating and drinking events toward activities, such as bowling, dancing, roller skating, or spectator sports.
- Allow more time for meal preparation and enjoyment. Rushed dinners are likely to contain quickie carbohydrates and fast fries.
- Rest frequently, sleep longer. Be active but avoid long periods of heavy mental or physical work that cause fatigue. Fatigue is an eater's pitfall.

If you can avoid these food oriented pitfalls, you are disconnecting a few of the "bells" that otherwise send out a false appetite cry.

If you can think of a few additional pitfalls, problem oriented to what you have discovered about yourself, more dinner bells will stop ringing.

As the false appetite bells stop ringing, you may eventually hear your real hunger sound loud and clear for the first time in years.

NOW PLACE A FEW PITFALLS IN THE
WAY OF IMPROPER EATING

My patients make excellent psychologists.

They have devised ingenious ways to steer their thoughts away from food.

Here are a number of useful pitfalls they have placed between themselves and a dish of whatever. If I were overweight, I would use many of them:

- Enjoy television, radio or hi-fi.
- Read the newspapers and magazines.
- Change the subject, if food comes up in a conversation.
- Phone your stock broker. Chit chat with a friend.
- Make love. Make any kind of joy.
- Count to 100. Count your money. Count your blessings.
- Take a look in a full length mirror. Observe areas needing improvement.
- Take a shower, or soak in the tub. Take a swim.
- Look out the window. Daydream. Star gaze. Meditate.
- Drink water, decaffeinated coffee or other permitted beverage. Chew gum (sugarless).
- Ride a bike or a horse or take a drive.
- Play the piano, a harmonica, etc. Sing or hum a tune.
- Water the lawn. Trim the flowers. Enjoy nature.
- Go to a library. Read a book (this one?).

- Go to a health club, gym or sauna.
- Take a course. Find a job. Become involved.
- Visit a friend. Go to the park or a concert.
- Walk the dog. Walk the kids. Take a hike.
- Paint, sew, crochet, knit, etc.
- Do an errand. Do a good deed. Do good. Do.
- Do calisthenics. Walk. Run.

Some of these useful pitfalls will work for you.

The thing is—something will work for you, if you work.

Be creative. Or just be. Do something on the spur of the moment that trips you up before you gather too much momentum toward the kitchen or lunch counter.

Here is something I want you to do. Do it before bedtime:

HOW TO: REINFORCE SUCCESSFUL METHODS

When you are in bed, ready to go to sleep, think about the day's events. Check your failures about improper eating. Where did you go wrong? Now check your successes. Congratulate yourself on them. Note these successes well. See yourself relying on these successful methods again whenever necessary.

HOW TO WORK OFF A FALSE APPETITE
OTHER THAN BY CHEWING AND SWALLOWING

It is not necessarily true that exercise burns less calories while it stimulates hunger for many more. In fact, strenuous exercise before a meal frequently acts to decrease one's hunger for that meal.

Exercise is a classic method of sublimation, to convert basic physical needs into an acceptable activity. Adolescents are encouraged to take part in sports to channel excessive energy for improved health. Certainly there is great merit in exercise to sublimate impulsive eating as well.

There are many exercises my patients enjoy doing as they slim down. Exercise in spare moments, whenever and wherever appropriate. Or at such strategic times as

Before a meal
Before a coffee break
Before a snack.

Don't think of exercises as calorie burners. View them instead as:

- Tension easers
- Boredom breakers
- Eating urge interrupters
- Muscle toners
- Limber uppers
- Emotional releasers

Don't give exercises an exclusive connection with the urge to eat. Enjoy them for themselves.

DEMOTE FOOD FROM A REWARD STATUS

If you are a parent, you know how easy it is to promise your youngster a cookie or a piece of candy providing he behaves. He does, and the reward is bestowed. It probably happened to you when you were a child.

When this happens again and again, food becomes more than food for the stomach. It becomes food for the ego, food for starving emotions, food for attention.

The pacifier used with infants today may save wear and tear on the thumb but free of calories as it may be, it still reinforces oral gratification as a reward.

Parents soon switch from pacifier to food. Food is a reward for good marks at school, for helping mother with the dishes and for just staying out of the way. It's also used as a reward for eating.

"No dessert unless you clean your plate."

Do you feel the need to reward yourself? For example having lost two pounds this week? Have a piece of pie, just this once. (Just this once contains enough carbohydrate calories to hang three pounds of fat on you with some help from other foods.)

Seldom do we give a child a piece of steak as a reward. It's usually a piece of cake, pie or other sweet.

The rewards of liquor are somewhat different. Burdens are lifted temporarily and we enjoy a brief euphoria. Unfortunately we pay the price for this sooner or later.

But focusing upon rewarding children with sweets, there are two unhappy outcomes:

1. Fat cells are produced in the young child which remain through adolescence and into adulthood. These fat cells may shrink at times of weight loss, yet remain ready to expand readily again at the drop of a hot fudge sundae. Children rewarded constantly with sweets are actually being primed for obesity.

2. Sweets are conditioned as a symbol of love—mother's love, father's love, self-love.

Did you sell a new account today? How about a dinner treat tonight?

Did you finish that project finally? How about stopping at the bakery on your way home?

Did you work hard? Tired? How about an ice cream soda?

Is there a way to answer no? Yes.

You can decondition yourself away from sweets or other food as a reward.

You can recondition yourself to accept some replacement as an equally satisfying reward.

It's as easy as sitting in a chair, relaxing, and giving yourself instructions to switch rewards.

I will explain this procedure in step-by-step detail in Chapter 8. I will share the techniques that can work quickly and effectively for you.

Meanwhile, you can begin by thinking about pleasurable activities you may use to reward yourself in place of food.

Some of my patients have used:

- Buying a new book
- Going to a movie or show
- Taking an overnight or weekend trip
- Treating to a new suit, dress, sport outfit, accessory, etc.
- Going to a gym, masseur, sauna or steam bath
- Visiting the beauty parlor or barber shop
- Chewing a stick of no-cal gum

Others have taken to food substitution, continuing food as a reward but limited to high protein, low fat, low carbohydrate items:

- A steak
- A turkey
- A low-cal soda

- A gelatin or custard dessert
- A program oriented snack

THE BIGGEST PITFALL OF ALL—CRAVING

"I crave chocolate. I just love it. I don't know why. I think it will go away. But it doesn't. I would rather have a candy bar than a whole meal. I think about the chocolate and my salivary glands start to squirt juices. Isn't your body supposed to dry out from such a craving, so you don't think about it anymore?"

If I closed my eyes I could see a child in my office. But this was a 50-year-old woman who had lost only three of her 157 pounds in two months. I now understand why.

"Craving is a subconscious conditioning that you must recondition or reprogram," I explained. "You can make chocolate taste like sour pickles if you really desire to eliminate the craving."

She reassured me she did. I helped her to understand the relaxation procedure. Then I instructed her about which image to visualize in her mind to accomplish the reprograming.

It was an image of chocolate turning to fat as it trickled down her throat.

This proved to be enough. The image soon became very repulsive. She could forego chocolate very easily after only three self-reprograming sessions.

Some patients will kill themselves with an overload of fat rather than divulge their craving:

"I don't know why I am not losing. I'm not a compulsive eater. The girls at work eat everything including candy. I don't. My husband and I eat the same foods, except he eats breakfast and I don't. He eliminated sugar and lost 25 pounds. I don't use sugar. Here I am with a wardrobe full of clothes I can't wear."

"What do you intend to do about it?" I asked this 55-year-old woman who worked at accounting and was aware of what 40 pounds of excess weight did to figures.

"I'm tense. I have a lot of problems at home. I cannot stay on a 500-calorie diet. When I'm nervous I'm unhappy and depressed. I don't love myself. I think about my husband—he doesn't make enough for us. My mother lives with us and nags constantly. I go on eating binges, eat at odd times and stuff myself with fattening foods. Like chocolate cookies and cake, but only a little bit."

Finally, she put her finger on it.

The subconscious likes to protect its cravings. As ingenious as the alcoholic can be hiding the bottle, the cake eater and the chocolate eater can be twice so. Today, at a slimmer 135 pounds, our woman accountant readily admits to secret hiding places for coffee cakes and brownies, layer cakes and Danish pastries.

Sometimes a craving masquerades as a necessity:

> "I have discovered one thing about myself. Some people smoke when they are nervous. I eat. The icebox seems to calm my nerves. Especially bread. I don't consider myself a nervous person, but whenever I become nervous, instead of crying or smoking I eat bread. It soothes my nerves. I love bread and can eat a whole sour dough loaf with butter. Mother makes it for me all the time."

Of course this 25-year old young married had to do a little more thinking about herself and her yen for bread. Once she did she was able to recognize the craving, not as a sedative she thought it to be, but a Pavlov bell—a programed response that needed reprograming.

It is always a thrill to me to see breakthroughs in weight control—both on and off the scale.

> I never scowled once at R.S., although weeks passed without losing a pound. A weight loss from 132 to 121 in four months is not exactly a miracle, but measured in other changes it was just that.
>
> Here was a woman, 56, who had not dated once in the six years since her divorce. She admitted she felt like something discarded. Her attitude changed ten times as much as her weight. She literally became a person again, joined a club, met a man and was having a ball.

> R.B., 42, did not lose any weight to speak of—from 145 to 137 in six weeks. But she went from: "I'm miserable, I hate myself, I've tried everything so I'll try your program."—to: "My marriage has turned great, I love myself, I feel like a mother to my little girl instead of a grandmother."
>
> Does it really matter how many pounds, how fast? R.B. is going to eliminate her weight problem for good and control her life.

> It's of little concern who you are, what you are doing, or when in life you make the decision. Decide to be conscious about your own consciousness and you rocket yourself to a superior life.

V.I. was a bookkeeper's bookkeeper. You know the type: thick rimmed glasses, no make-up, long skirts, outdated hairdo. She appeared closer to 50 than 36. At 169, she was almost 40 pounds overweight for her 5'6" frame.

Her husband was the opposite type: handsome, outgoing, a successful real estate salesman. He was seeing other women. V.I. eventually learned about this. First, she went the nervous breakdown route, then decided this wasn't going to help.

"My competition was a good-looking girl. I decided to lose weight—not for him,—for me." She shed 24 pounds in less than two months. Then she began wearing make-up, a new hairdo, modern large multi-colored plastic eyeglasses, and fashionable clothes. She enrolled in business courses at night. Soon he had to run to catch up to her. But he couldn't run fast enough. She found her own apartment, led her own life.

HALF WAY SUM UP

You are now at the half way point in this book. I bring this to your attention because I remember my friend saying to me I wouldn't be able to help my readers perform weight and self-programing miracles such as my patients have done.

I want you to help me prove him wrong. I want you to begin thinking about your life and about you.

I want you to pinpoint problems, identify those false appetite triggers we have been calling "Pavlov's bells," examine your own opinions of yourself, and spotlight pitfalls.

List all problems.

appetite triggers
negative self-opinions
and eating pitfalls.

We will work on this list together in Chapter 8, programing out the eroding effect of problems, the appetite stimulation of "bells," the need for stomach building as ego bolstering, and the attraction of program pitfalls.

But first, in Chapter 7, I want to let you know what a wonderful person you really are.

It is important that you know.

The Meat of Chapter 6

Ask yourself, "What pitfalls are my undoing?" List the ideas that come to you about your life—home, business, social—which affect your eating habits.

Begin an intensive mind-body program with the ten "Just for Today" commandments. Visualize yourself complying with each one in turn. This visualizing is subtle reprograming. It works!

Identify the pitfalls you want to avoid—the appetite triggers, the thoughts and problems that sap your self-esteem, the cravings. List them for future reprograming sessions you will be doing in Chapter 8.

Meanwhile, throw a few obstacles in the way of your false appetites and fattening cravings, such as an activity or an exercise.

7

HOW TO DEVELOP A MENTAL "SET" THAT PROGRAMS YOU FOR SLENDERIZING SUCCESS

Appetizer for Chapter 7

You cannot go anywhere unless you know your destination and you set a course. Chapter 7 is not exactly an automatic pilot, or even a roadmap. But it tells you where to find and how to use—both.

Thin people live longer than fat people.

In a recent issue of Soviet Woman, a leading Russian magazine, the question of how to postpone the onset of old age was discussed. As a rule, thin people live longer in Russia, too. They suffer less from illness and from arteriosclerosis.

Three other major factors contributing to aging also noted were insufficient exercise, emotional stress and environmental forces or pollutants. The Russians pinpointed sugar as one of the chief dietary threats to health. They plugged foods rich in minerals and vitamins as aids to long life.

I am a bariatric physician. But I often feel like a gerontologist.

Bariatrics is devoted to weight control. Gerontology is devoted to life extension.

Their routes coincide much of the way.

Exercise, peace of mind and lots of fresh air are part of my clinical program, too. They all pay off in the beautification of figures, feelings and faces.

Would you like to guess which is the most popular game in the United States? The answer—Russian Roulette.

Over one-third of all the men and women in our country are pointing the pistol of death due-to-overweight at themselves and gambling that it won't happen to them.

Overweight people need more oxygen when they are resting. This means the heart also pumps harder when they are sleeping. Of course, when they are working the added work load on the heart is greater. Overweight increases the resistance of blood vessels to blood flow. The left ventricle of the heart takes on the task.

Next time you look in the mirror, make a promise to your left ventricle.

SET A GOAL IN POUNDS OR INCHES

"Obesity is an insidious killer that affects both the body and spirit of its victims."

The speaker is Dr. B.D. Howland addressing the American Society of Bariatric Physicians on accepting its presidency in November, 1972. He used this occasion to exhort attending physicians to advance bariatric medicine so that the more than 60 million obese and overweight people in this country can enjoy successful treatment.

Dr. Howland called these 60 million "the most ignored silent majority." In my office they are far from silent.

They talk.

They cry.

They write.

They phone.

I know with every word comes understanding of self and a restoration of normality—in weight and in health.

However, somewhere along the way, and the sooner the better, a weight loss goal needs to be set.

As you approach your optimum weight, miraculous changes occur. You don't have to step on a scale to know you are making progress.

Here's how one woman describes the changes she experienced:

"An inner glow seems to radiate and permeate my surroundings. The feeling of well-being which energizes me increases ten-fold with each passing week. My body is lighter and more flexible.

"The skin on my legs, for instance, after a day of activity would become tight and stretched by the bloating or swelling in the tissues. Now, with a reduction in the size of my calves, my skin is softer and more elastic, but firm.

"Also, the pores of my skin seem to be smaller in size and less troublesome to keep clean. Bulges, here and there, are being flattened by exercise and the visual effect is a bonus to my emotional health."

As F.B., 34, mother of three, reached her 118 goal, less than six months after weighing in at 155, here's how she described the beneficial changes:

"With loss of weight I noticed many physical improvements—less stiffness of the knees (I have a trick knee and am especially conscious of aches or stiffness in that joint), diminution of cramps and aches in the legs after being on my feet all day, complete elimination of shortness of breath after running upstairs or doing heavy physical exertion.

"Loss of weight eliminated most of my fatigue, contributed to increased endurance during physical activity and enabled me to accomplish more without becoming overly tired. I noticed beneficial effects on my skin—a mild case of acne cleared, there is a healthier glow to my skin and less splotchiness of my complexion. I haven't been bothered by headaches, and infrequent backaches were eliminated completely. Stomach flatulence disappeared.

"My appearance improved very much. I lost a large amount of flab and reduced my clothing almost two sizes. Many commented on how much younger I appeared after losing more than 20 pounds!

"Weight loss has enabled me to meet others without undue self-consciousness about looking fat. I feel more relaxed and at ease. I am more cheerful and feel happier about myself. Through meditation I am more aware of why I eat, of all sorts of occurrences which tend to make me eat for reasons other than true hunger. I was able to stop myself and ask 'Are you eating because you're truly hungry?' "

Why do I call this book a "miracle" guide? I think this patient has supplied the answer in her letter to me. Many patients have accomplished similar miracles in this program. The miracle may take one of several forms and may vary in degree.

Some patient's ultimate weight goals are higher than other's overweight starting points. Do you think someone weighing 189 needs to drop a few pounds? Perhaps you're right. But W.G. dropped 135 of her pounds to reach 189, having started on the program at a mammoth 324. Of course, she should lose more, and maybe she did later, but I congratulated her at the end of 7½ months for a job well done.

Here is my staff's description of her "before" and "after":

BEFORE—Sloppy dress, body odor, no make-up, withdrawn, cries all the time, gray hair roots showing, nervous, depressed, suicidal, tired, dizzy spells.
AFTER—New clothes, dyed hair, fragrantly alluring, make-up, talks with patients about how great she feels, more energetic, dating, married, brought wedding pictures in for display.

A man quit at 183 pounds after losing 103 pounds. W.E., 27, was a computer programer so he knew how to program himself into healthful eating habits. He ate five or six times a day, only small amounts of high protein foods. He knew he could succeed because he had come into the program a few years before, fearful he would be drafted if he lost too much weight. This time he stayed with it 18 months. Here is his "before" and "after":

BEFORE—Sloppy, not friendly, hypertension, tired, introverted.
AFTER—Dressing in double knits, sociable, blood pressure normal, energetic, brought in girl friend, stopped smoking, married.

"What is my best weight?"
"What measurements do I wish to attain?"
One or both of these questions must be answered with conviction and enthusiasm. The answer can then be recorded on a graph to indicate your progress.

Some physicians require a date as part of the weight loss goal. I don't. You're going to be slender the rest of your life. Taking several weeks or a few months more or less of time is unimportant, just so you eventually reach your goal.

These best measurements or best weight goals must be realistic. A 6' man cannot aim for 130 pounds, or 5'10" woman 110 pounds. Your own physician can advise you about your best weight and/or measurements.

You shed pounds on this program wherever excess fat occurs.

B.J. at 18 weighed 156 pounds. At 5'8" she didn't look heavy. But she had the legs of an elephant. It required five months to drop 24 pounds and it all came off from her thighs downward. Extra dividends: B.J. always wore jeans, hardly talked, let her long dishwater blonde hair fall in all directions. Now she wears short dresses, and short shag styled hair. She talked a mile a minute about her travels and her new boy friends. And she stopped smoking.

There is more to setting a goal than meets the eye.

Although you are setting a physical goal, you are also creating a mental "set."

The very act of setting a goal starts you on a journey. The goal is your destination. When you drive to the store or work or home, you often find you're there before you realize. Perhaps you were thinking about how to make a sale or a date, but your subconscious mind knew where you wanted to go and unconsciously helped make all the turns.

When you set a weight goal, you are programing yourself for daily behavior that will help to lead you to these goals.

I say "help." You need more programing than to merely set a goal—as you well know.

Take Dianne. She weighed somewhat over 300 pounds. Her goal was 120. Now, after about two months she was 268. Then she met Tom:

"Wednesday night I met a marvelous man. We talked for three hours in a coffee shop. I gradually recognized the qualities of this man—his integrity, his self-assurance, his complete containment within himself, yet without conceit—a truly tremendous person.

"We made a date for Thursday and he was to pick me up at 7 p.m.

"He didn't show and he didn't call.

"Until now I was OK. There could be explanations.

"When Friday passed with still no word, my own private demons broke out and I fell apart.

"I began to feel it was my fault. I wasn't good enough for him. I had bored him, etc., etc., etc.

"By Saturday morning, the fear began to set in. (This also was the *exact* day I had marked on my calendar to watch for the pre-menstrual tension, upset, etc.).

"Soon I was in limbo and fear had taken over completely. Tears started. I walked around the room and thought about things and again tears flowed. I slowly began to realize that the trigger point had been meeting Tom—it was unexpected and unplanned. I certainly felt more womanly and female as opposed to being a 'blob,' but I just wasn't prepared to meet a man I was truly attracted to. Anyway, here I was—still gargantuan and all of a sudden I met this incredible man whom I enjoyed thoroughly and who seemed to enjoy my company also.

"When he didn't show up for our date Thursday, I guess it was like seeing a bubble burst—it's gone and you're not sure how to make another one."

Needless to say, Dianne was primed for a return to 300 pounds when Tom broke the date. She was also aware of the effect her menstrual cycle could have on her emotions. More important, she was able to step back and look at herself while the drama was being played, as if she was the audience instead of the tragedienne.

Her goal helped to restore her emotions. Then her restored emotions helped to reprogram her goal. If there had been a few days of sorry-for-herself eating, they were quickly ended and the path to her goal was resumed. When I last saw her she weighed less than one-half her weight since her first visit.

People set goals every day and never reach them.

Most diet books advise you to set a goal in the first few chapters. I have resisted until more than half way through this book. Even now, I do so with reservations.

If you set goals and attain them, you program yourself for success.

Starvation and crash diets are doomed to end in failure of one sort or another. So you pave the way for the next diet to end similarly.

I want you to set a goal. But I also want you to be so practiced at thinking about yourself and programing yourself correctly that you *must* and *will* reach your goal.

WHY YOU DO REACH YOUR GOAL IN THIS PROGRAM

Less than 5 percent of the people achieve their goals in life. The main reasons they fail are:

1. The goals are not clearly defined.
2. It is more a dream than a goal, with the dreamer knowing full well it cannot come true.
3. There is a willingness to settle for less.

If you can visualize your goal clearly . . .

If you can agree with yourself that it is rightfully yours . . .

If you can keep your goal in view despite temptations to settle for less . . .

. . . Claim it. It *is* yours.

Can you visualize yourself weighing 25, 50, 100 pounds less, or whatever your goal is? Can you see yourself wearing smaller sizes? Can you see your mirror view, your side view, your back view? Can you see yourself coming closer week by week and finally arriving?

Can you accept this slender profile as the real *you*? Do you feel you have a right to be thin, attractive, popular? Can you see yourself as normally slender?

Suppose you succeed in approaching a goal, is that acceptable? Will you stop ten or fifteen pounds short, or maybe thirty or more if there is lots of poundage involved, and say, "Well, that's close enough." Or will you insist on going all the way?

For most diets, it's do or die, otherwise you don't succeed. The pain of the diet is insurmountable. If the motive is not titanic and the effort herculean, you usually settle for less or fail to reach your goal.

Not so on my program. It is designed to permit the average goalmaker to succeed without pain and with average motivation.

Instead of do or die, it's food and fun. The nonfattening food. Fun exploring human nature and turning grey clouds into pure sunlight. Fun working toward and achieving your goal.

YOUR CONSCIOUSNESS RUNS A REMARKABLE INSTRUMENT

Your body is a remarkable instrument. It makes the most intricate space station appear to be a toy.

This body of yours is a self-rebuilding machine. It maintains the same temperature within whether you are shivering in below zero weather or perspiring in tropical heat. It contains a furnace that uses any type fuel as food. It boasts a chemical laboratory that can create alkalies, acids and drugs so powerful that a single drop could poison a lake.

It has a pump that surpasses the most efficient man-made pump, a skeleton that is an engineering miracle, and a central computer containing billions of cells, able to operate the system perfectly.

There is just one hitch . . .

The central computer has someone doing its programing who is the best person available, yet not quite perfect at his job.

That person is you.

A perfect machine needs a perfect operator to make it work perfectly.

If the operator has self-doubts, family problems, sexual frustrations, feelings of self-recrimination . . . oops, wrong button pushed—too much acid, not enough blood sugar, low on adrenalin, etc.

Your consciousness is the key

If you are willing to let your consciousness ferret out its hang-ups and become weight goal oriented, you're much closer to achieving your goal.

Over two thousand years ago, one of history's wisest men, Socrates, said it in two words: "Know Thyself."

Once you become aware of your own thoughts, feelings, and emotions, you are a giant step closer to being their master.

Once you are the master of your own consciousness, every picture you hold in it, especially about yourself, is automatically produced by this remarkable computerized space ship you call your body.

THE CONNECTION BETWEEN A SLENDER GOAL
AND A POUND OF FAT

A Sonoma (California) State College Professor operates an Institute for the Treatment of Obesity and Overeating. Participants are urged to bring their favorite foods to one of the workshops. They then experience exactly why they enjoy those foods. Is it because they are soft and oozy, hot or cold, brittle and crunchy?

The different food awareness exercises help people to discover where they feel hunger (jaw, mouth, neck, stomach, back, shoulder); which side of the mouth they favor (those who like the back of the mouth are encouraged to use a straw more frequently); and what emotions seem to dominate at the time of extra eating (anger, tension, loneliness, etc.).

Although I don't agree with all of the techniques, I do endorse the efforts to help participants become aware of their reactions to food.

This awareness becomes the connecting link between the mental and the physical.

The more you are aware of *you*—the emotions that trigger mouth hunger rather than stomach hunger, the foods you eat and the times you eat them, the right and the wrong foods for your health—the more the mental "set" we call a goal is able to reach its target: fat.

Recently the American Academy of Family Physicians heard a report on the results of a study of 21 men and women who had one thing in common: each weighed over 300 pounds. Held at The Georgetown University (Washington, D.C.) Medical Center and Hospital, the study showed a striking unawareness by these obese people of how much food they were actually eating.

"Doctor," says the obese patient, "I really don't know why I am fat. My meals are small. I eat like a bird."

A vulture, maybe?

After the participants became aware of what they were eating and why they were eating (hunger of the mind), they lost an average of 180 pounds each within six months.

When I ask you to set a goal, I'm not asking you to select weight and body measurements which make you look the best.

Vanity is fine. But it is not a very solid foundation to set, and reach, a weight goal.

When I ask you to set such a goal, I am asking you to set a goal for understanding yourself, for self-awareness, for self-acceptance.

If you are turned off about knowing yourself, you would have closed this book long ago. So I know we are walking this path of self-discovery together.

It is a great path.

The milestones that are ticked off are made of fat.

The goal is a great new life for slender you.

THE SHORT VIEW LEADS TO THE LONG VIEW

You begin to see a pattern in the changes which come over men and women. There are many. Here are ten I see frequently:

- Sloppiness turns to neatness.
- Old-fashioned eyeglasses turn modern or contact.
- Hair styles are changed—for the better.
- Clothing becomes more "in."
- Manner of standing becomes more erect.
- Manner of walking becomes more precise.
- Having a good time supersedes "the miseries."
- Non-talkative types become congenial and outgoing.
- Stagnation in social life yields to progress.
- Failures in business end, successes begin.

Here are some flashes in my "passing parade":

A.L., 45, divorcee, scaled herself down 16 pounds in six weeks and remarried her husband.

S.J., 48, 178 pounds, was worried about her husband's frequent business trips. She tossed away 38 pounds in six months and now he has been inviting her to travel with him.

L.G., 25, fighting diabetes for 10 years, dropped not only 25 pounds but her high blood sugar as well.

P.T., 37, an engineer, controlled his drinking along with his weight, and stopped smoking to boot.

S.B., 23, would sit in the office for hours as she had no one to talk to. When her weight dropped from 168 to 132 in three months, she began missing appointments due to her social whirl.

F.C., 52, at 143 pounds wouldn't talk to anyone or reply when spoken to. Four months later, weighing 118, she was calling everybody "dear," including me.

D.P., 38, the real estate sales agent, appeared intent on proving she could also be a yo-yo on my program. She has been in and out of the program five times, losing and regaining an average of 30 pounds. I will be seeing her again.

D.L., 22, hid her pimpled face behind big sunglasses and her 198 pounds inside a coat. When she reached 164 her complexion improved. Then she bought sets of different colored contact lenses to match her many shades of eye make-up. And the coat disappeared.

S.L., 33, a sloppily dressed social worker, lived in a slum area and really looked the part. When she slimmed down, her appearance improved, she dressed mod and moved to a neighborhood more in keeping with her upgraded self.

Don't settle for less as you achieve your weight loss goal. Meanwhile, many important life problems will drift away on your seemingly miraculous journey.

The ultimate goal needs to be programed into your subconscious mind (techniques discussed in the next chapter), then mostly forgotten in favor of the day-to-day program.

I see so many patients who want to give up because the goal seems so far away. I urge them not to look at the long range goal. It can appear to be an overwhelming task.

Instead of looking so far down the road, take the program one day at a time, knowing that each day brings you closer to understanding yourself, closer to disconnecting emotional appetite bells, closer to adopting permanently correct eating habits, closer to your long range goal of attractiveness.

Yes, the program programs you. Couple this type of behavior programing with automatic mind-body programing (Chapter 8), and the results are smooth sailing and effortless, permanent weight and fat loss.

Here are daily goals:

HOW TO: YOUR GOAL FOR TODAY

- To eat proper, high protein, high nutrition foods.
- To be aware of my eating and to extract as much enjoyment as possible from each savoured mouthful.
- To be aware of my emotions, attitudes and feelings so I can substitute the positive, wholesome, and happy for the negative, sapping and sad.
- To jot down the discoveries about my emotions, attitudes and feelings prior to, during and after eating or the impulse to eat.
- To have at least one programing session (using the techniques in the next chapter).
- To be active in mind as well as in body.

"What? No pounds-off and inches-off goals?" you ask.

"No," I reply. "Fulfill these five daily goals and the pounds and inches will take care of themselves."

Do it. You will see. You will achieve.

THE IMPORTANCE OF THIS VERY MOMENT TO YOU

I would propose an even shorter dimension in setting goals.

Your long range goal measured in terms of your optimum weight (decided by you and your physician) or in terms of your tape measure readings may require weeks, months, or even longer, depending on your personal situation.

Your daily goal requires 24 hours.

How about a moment-to-moment goal? It requires only a second.

Ask yourself, "Where am I at this very moment?"

It is where you are at this very moment that is important. What can you learn now, do now, experience now? What you accomplish this moment determines whether you will ride, fly, or soar the next moment—or become sidetracked in the kitchen.

Spend this moment thinking about yourself. Here are a few questions to start your thoughts moving. If one tugs at you, let it.

HOW TO: THOUGHTS FOR A
PERSONAL RAP SESSION

"Why am I important?"

"What does this weight control program mean to me?"

"Do I love me?"

"What is in a lifetime beside eating, sleeping, and making love?"

"What did I eat last and why?"

"Can success come to (your name)?"

"What worry, anxiety or concern is in the back of my mind at this moment and how can I re-assure myself?"

Now I am not suggesting you go from moment to moment thinking about yourself and let the rest of the world go by.

It would be great, though—great for you—if you would stop every now and then to have such a rap session. Pick your times strategically. Let them block impulse eating.

Make these moments count.

THE SECRET INGREDIENT IN EVERY INSTANCE
OF A GOAL SUCCESSFULLY REACHED

We have talked about three types of weight loss goals:

1. The weight or measurement goal.
2. The daily goal.
3. The moment-by-moment goal.

There is a fourth. It has nothing to do with weight control. Yet has everything to do with it:

4. The life goal.

How can any goal succeed if a person is drifting in life?

It may come as a shock to you that you are here on a mission.

Now mission is a fairly high sounding word. "I'm not a Florence Nightingale or a Henry Kissinger," you say.

But you are who you are.

There is no one else the same as you in the entire world. There is no one with your exact abilities, proclivities, competence, gifts, qualifications, endowments, learnings, skills, and special approach.

Everyone's mission is to assist other people. You fit into the activities of people in a very special way. Here are some possible activities:

- You may have a knack growing food or flowers, or caring for animals.
- You may be a good listener and help people who need to vent their problems.
- You may be able to concentrate on details such as are needed in an office or factory.
- You may have a desire for cleanliness and are better able than others to clean, straighten and restore order out of disorder.
- You may have a natural ability to help others dress and look their best.
- You may have a way of seeing behind a forest of detail and knowing what must be done.
- You may be great at preparing and serving food.
- You may be able to program your mind to type on typewriters, to operate office machines, or to program electronic computers.
- You may be able to understand and assist children to learn and grow.
- You may be able to create a home base for a man or woman, enabling them to better carry out their mission.

These are only ten activities. Life includes countless types of missions. They are as important as the higher sounding types of missions, such as an inventor, scientist, nurse, doctor, lawyer, clergyman, philosopher, poet, astronaut, writer, sportsman, actor, etc.

There is a place for everyone—except the person who thinks, and consequently programs himself, that he has no place.

A hospital nearby hired an in-patient interviewer. Hospitals don't usually want a Marilyn Monroe type for this job. They were safe with V.L., a neatly dressed, buxom woman of 52. Little did they know she had just embarked on our weight control program.

In six months, she could just as well have been a fashion model—svelte at the waist, she flaunted an hour-glass figure that attracted many glances.

Doctors and interns stopped to chat with her. Ambulatory male patients beat a path to her desk.

Her home life was a joy. "My husband is delighted with my weight loss and attitude. We're on a honeymoon every day." When her son married, many thought she was the bride.

And the hospital was happy, too. She was good for morale.

What can you do if you are a professional ice skater and you gain 50 pounds? G.C. decided that if she didn't lose those pounds pronto, she could eventually become a comic skater. She certainly could make them laugh in her bulging tights. One month into the program she identified the reason for her affinity with pastries, and reprogramed pastries out of her life. When she hit 111 on the scales, she was skating for hours on end and in the prime of her career. And she noticed some side effects—all good: her legs didn't ache anymore, she was no longer a borderline diabetic. Now she sends joke books about fat people for my office.

How can a slenderizing goal succeed if there is no life goal into which it can fit?

You are unique. You have a special mission. Do you know what it is?

If you do, you are ready to proceed.

If you don't know your life goal, you can discover it now.

It is in your mind. All you have to do is let it out of the subconscious where it has been buried and permit it to enter the conscious mind.

How do you do this? Just as you would any other thoughts you wish to retrieve from the subconscious.

Remember the last time you couldn't put your finger on someone's name? It was almost on the tip of your tongue but you couldn't quite grab it. So you stopped thinking about it. Then it popped into your mind—perhaps minutes or hours later.

Do this with your life goal or mission.

You knew it once, perhaps many years ago. Recall it. If you don't, then relax. Maybe a few minutes or hours later, it will pop into your mind. Perhaps while you're shaving or cooking. "Oh," you'll say, "of course—that's it!"

HOW TO: REMEMBER YOUR LIFE GOAL

Set the book down. Ask yourself, "Now, let me see, what is my life goal?" Continue reading, or doing other things. The answer will arrive.

When the answer does arrive, shake hands with yourself. Welcome yourself back to the human race.

You are now ready to embark on the program with a course set. Like a ship's captain, you have received your orders. You have set a course to reach the ordered destination, with appropriate ports along the way. You have stocked the ship with high protein, high mineral, high vitamin foods. The tide of enthusiasm is rising.

Bon Voyage!

The Meat of Chapter 7

Set a specific weight goal in pounds off, or a specific measurement goal in inches off. Accept the goal as real, claim it as rightfully yours. Set a day-to-day goal for eating properly, thinking, understanding, writing, programing. Be aware of yourself at critical moments, as a minute-to-minute type of goal. But above all, remind yourself of your life goal. Set all goals as spelled out in the "How To" sections.

8

END FAULTY EATING HABITS,
BEGIN SLENDERIZING HABITS
PRACTICALLY INSTANTLY
WITH SELF-HYPNOSIS

Appetizer for Chapter 8

Pavlov's appetite bells ringing in your stomach, frustrations driving you to food and drink, cycles of ups and downs.

Kiss them all good-bye.

This is the big moment. You now learn how to turn off what you don't need, turn on what you do need.

The effect is that you no longer want what you don't need. Can you ask for anything more?

Pavlov trained his dogs to salivate on the ringing of a bell only after many conditionings or programings. He would ring the bell and provide them with food scores and scores of times before the bell finally began to signal food and activate the saliva.

If Pavlov were able to talk to the dogs, he could have limited the whole procedure to a few days instead of several months.

Here's what he would say, "Relax, Fidovitch. Close your eyes. Be quiet and peaceful. Now, when I ring this bell, imagine your dinner has arrived."

If Fidovitch cooperated, it could require only three such sessions and that bell would bring the dog's saliva a-drooling.

Pavlov could not talk to his dogs in this manner. However, you can talk to yourself this way.

If you cooperate, you can do the same thing in reverse within a few days. You can reprogram yourself so that certain times on the clock no longer ring an appetite bell for you, also certain personal events won't do it, and anything that has been triggering your salivary glands or your thoughts of eating when you are not actually hungry will be de-fused.

Let's make one thing clear right now: If all you do is continue on the high protein-low fat and low carbohydrate program in Chapter 3, you will shed weight and fat. If you also think and write about yourself, that is better yet, and you are increasing the probability that you will never regain the weight and fat you shed.

However, only the reconditioning you are about to learn now can make continuing on the program effortless and remaining slender always a foregone conclusion.

THE SERVO-MECHANISM THAT, UNFORTUNATELY, YOU SERVE

When you learn to type or play the piano or drive a car, you practice. Then you are able to do it.

"Practice" means repetition.

"Do it" means function automatically without hardly having to think about it.

Repetition enables you to function automatically. It makes typing or playing the piano or driving the car almost as undemanding of your conscious effort as breathing.

What is happening is that repetition is programing your subconscious mind. This subconscious mind is the automatic part of the mind. Program it thoroughly and it follows your programing without question.

It is a servo-mechanism.

The problem is that the subconscious accepts programing through repetition whether it is repeated practice sessions on a typewriter or repeated eating sessions at a table. It is programed by repetition whether you want it to be or not.

It would be a fantastic life if we could sit at the table and turn off our servomechanism. "I'm eating. But this time it's off the record."

We cannot turn off that automatic part of our mind. It is turned on with birth, off with death. In between, everything acts as programing with repetition adding emphasis.

As a result, you are the servant of your servomechanism, instead of the way it should be. It directs you most of the time instead of you directing it.

This is why you are overweight.

Sure, it's the apple turnovers and the plum puddings, the pretzels and the potato chips—because repetition, which you have permitted, has programed them into your subconscious mind.

If you play a musical instrument, you know how difficult it is to play a sour note. The comedian who deliberately plays a wrong note has had to work at it. It doesn't come easy. When the servomechanism is programed a certain way, carrying out that program is its function and your conscious mind can seldom successfully intervene.

Frankly, Mr. and Mrs. Overweight, your only hope is reprograming.

Continue on the program long enough and you will reprogram that servomechanism.

But the key is "long enough."

It's three o'clock—the servomechanism orders cake and coffee.
Damn this job!—the servomechanism orders two bottles of beer.
Where is he (or *she*)?—the servomechanism orders chocolate, ten minutes worth.

Can you resist? Of course not.
But you can reprogram so easily.
So very, very easily.

THE TWO SIMPLE STEPS TO END OVEREATING

Remember how I described Pavlov's mythical conversation with his dogs? "Relax . . . Imagine."

These are the two steps which reach into your servomechanism with new programing.

Sound easy? It is. But there's no fooling around here.

If you are not fully relaxed in body and mind, the entry into your servomechanism is not fully opened.

If you do not visualize as clearly as you can see a red watermelon, pits and all, new programing is not actually being fed into the servomechanism.

So you must relax profoundly in body and mind, more profoundly and completely than you are accustomed to doing.

It is fun. It is easy. I will show you how in this chapter.

You must spell out your proper new programing with positive words and realistic images.

This too is fun and easy and I will show you how.

Before I do, I want you once again to visit my office and eavesdrop at the door. I want you to listen to people talking to me about their conscious feelings and evaluations about eating improperly.

Most of all listen to their resolutions, words which mean "I will try." Will they succeed without reprograming? Can they possibly change their habits despite the most sincere intentions without reprograming? (The comments in parenthesis are my own):

"After I had my children, my weight went up and down all the time." (Why all the time?)

"One time I ate a dozen doughnuts. I could hardly believe it and didn't even realize it." (Do you know what events occurred or what your emotional state was at that time?)

"I'm just eating my way through life." (What are your reasons?)

"My husband and 16-year old boy eat anything and everything. They are both very slender. (What are the reasons you compete with them knowing you readily gain weight?)

"No one likes to be fat. I don't want to do anything when I'm fat. I don't look or feel good and my clothes look 'cruddy' on me." (Apparently you have been overweight many years. Why haven't you done something about it before?)

"I'm a nervous person, a compulsive eater." (According to whom and compared to what?)

"I don't know what I want. I know I'm like this but I don't know why. I was different when I lived in England. My family protected me. I was near people who cared about me." (Do you care about yourself?)

"Stuffing myself with food is an escape." (An escape from what?)

"My two small sons drive me batty so all I can do is eat. When they grow up I think it will be a different situation because we can exchange ideas and get out more often." (Will your sons help you with your weight problem?)

"I don't know which way to turn. I'm making every effort and no matter which way I turn there are no results. It's like running my head into a brick wall all the time." (Describe what you mean by a brick wall?)

"My husband can't discuss our problems with me. I try to please him but everything I do is wrong." (Can you tell me about things you do that you know are right?)

"I've had the habit of overeating for more than twenty years." (Are you suggesting you can't change the habit?)

"It seems that recently the weight goes on me much faster and in larger amounts. I think it's a matter of self-discipline. Eating is a luxury; if I can afford to eat, I do so." (Do you really think eating is a luxury?)

"I guess I will restrict myself, I will stick to the program, I will make a promise to myself and not anyone else." (Aren't these promises very often broken?)

"I realize I have an eating problem. I can last two days on the program, then I'm famished for other foods. (What do you mean by being famished?) I have an appetite or craving. It's merely lack of willpower, I know that." (What do you mean by willpower?)

"One part of me cares and one part doesn't care. One part wants to be young looking, slim, early thirties, the really vain part; the other part wants to be just frumpy, dumpy, middle-aged, grey haired, mother type. (Why?) I don't know; maybe I'm getting lazy. I eat more to feel better, then I feel worse, so I eat more to feel better again. Now my life is changing and I'm into middle age." (Why should this disturb you?)

"I lived a very sheltered, insulated life. Whenever I ran into trouble, I never had to take my own knocks. (What did you expect when you began this program?) Maybe I expected you to wave the magic wand, give me magic pills so I would be thin again."

These people needed to know techniques to relax.

They needed to know what images and words to use to reprogram themselves.

So do you.

Here goes.

THE SCIENCE AND ART OF REPROGRAMING
YOUR SERVO-MECHANISM

Remember the two steps? Relax. Visualize.

There are a number of techniques now in use to quiet the body and mind. I will explain a few to you. All you need is one—one that works best for you.

It's actually the mind that needs to be quiet and tranquil. But you cannot enjoy peace of mind if your body is tense or in an uncomfortable position.

I can hear your questions. "Suppose I fall asleep?" "Will I be able to end my relaxation?" "Suppose the baby should cry while I'm doing this?"

The answers should put all your fears to rest: If you fall asleep, it is the same as a regular nap. You awaken as you have done in the past whenever you have dozed.

You end your relaxation session anytime you decide.

You are quite aware while relaxed, able to respond more quickly than you would if you were absorbed in viewing television or listening to the radio.

There is no magic to this. Relaxing the body permits the conscious mind to relax. By relaxing the conscious mind, you are removing the sentry standing at the doorway to your subconscious mind or servomechanism. The sentry's name is Critical Faculty.

Your Critical Faculty needs to be temporarily withdrawn in order for programing to go directly to your servomechanism without any watering down and consequently without requiring constant repetition.

Let us continue with the science of relaxing. Here are three techniques:

I. Breathing technique

II. Eye technique

III. Head-to-toe technique

Let me first describe these to you one at a time. No need to do them now.

I. Breathing Technique. Sit comfortably in a straight back chair, legs uncrossed, hands on lap. Take a deep breath and as you exhale, let your eyes close gently. Take a second deep breath and feel your body relaxing from head to toe. Now take a third deep breath. Make it a real deep end-of-the-day sigh and let all your worries and problems be expelled with the air. Sit quietly for a few minutes, allowing your attention to dwell comfortably on your breathing. Feel yourself becoming more and more peaceful and tranquil with every breath you take.

II. Eye Technique. Sit comfortably as before. Stare at a point on your hand. Don't allow the eyes to blink. When, in a few moments, you feel the need to blink, let your eyes close gently. Let your attention dwell comfortably on your eyes. Be aware of every little sensation in your eye muscles. Coax your eye muscles to relax to the nth degree of perfect comfort. If the eyelids flutter or the eyes water, this is a good sign that your eyes are responding to your instructions. Once delightfully relaxed, send the feeling in them—the liquid comfort—like a wave down your body and all the way to your toes.

III. Head-to-Toe Technique. Sit comfortably as in the previous methods. Let your eyes close gently and permit your attention to drift to your scalp. Check out your scalp for tenseness. Permit the little muscles that control the scalp to relax. When you are sure your scalp muscles are not taut but are comfortably adjusted, do the same for your forehead. No furrows. No wrinkles. Perfectly smooth. Now your eyes. They may water or your eyelids may flutter. Consider these good signs. How do your face muscles feel? Your mouth? Is your tongue comfortable in your mouth? Perhaps your mouth will water or maybe you will feel the need to swallow. Again, these are good signs. Now move on down to your neck, shoulders, chest. Your arms should feel heavy on your lap. Maybe one feels heavier than the other. Or perhaps you don't know exactly where your arms are. All good signs. Now relax your stomach, hips, back, thighs, legs, feet, toes. You are now thoroughly relaxed from head to toe.

Each of these three methods are very successful. It is difficult to say which is better than the other. It can be decided either from the description or by checking each out.

Also, you can use any one, two, or all three, if you wish. If you do combine them, arrange them in this order:

II, I

or II, III

or I, III

or II, I, III

These are the scientific techniques for relaxation.
But relaxation of body and mind is also an art.

THE ART OF COOPERATING WITH YOURSELF

"Doctor, how can I be sure I am relaxed?" I hear that question so often.

Some people seem to expect a siren to go off when they reach a certain state of relaxation, or a bell to ring confirming that they are there.

This is no strange state to be in. You are there when you are watching a drama on television or sitting in a theater or just lying quietly in your favorite place of relaxation.

Accept your relaxation as accomplished.

Accept your visualizing as effective.

Accept the whole procedure as important to you.

Expect results.

The degree to which you can accept and expect is the degree to which you will be successful.

Psychologists call the two main ingredients of successful relaxation and programing—expectation and belief. Expectation is dependent on cooperation. Belief is dependent on acceptance.

Cooperate and accept.

MENTAL IMAGES THAT HELP EVERY TIME

Before you practice the three relaxation techniques, here, simply, are two ways to help feed new information into your mental computer or servomechanism. Why waste your first attempt at full relaxation? Why not use it to further your success in the program?

Pictures enter the subconscious and program it more effectively than words. Words work. But pictures work better.

The picture of you at your best weight is the picture you will be using most frequently in your daily periods of relaxation and imagining (visualizing).

You can use words, too. A Frenchman named Emil Coue made verbal programing popular earlier this century. We still hear, "Every day in every way I am getting better and better."

You can sit in your relaxed state and say short affirmations either aloud or to yourself. These statements then become true.

"I enjoy protein foods more and more every day. My tastes reflect my body's needs."

Repeat these words in your relaxed state and they become programing. They replace the sugar and starch programing that now impels your behavior.

In a few sessions of this programing you will be gravitating to the nonfattening foods as easily and naturally as you have in the past been attracted to the fattening foods.

YOUR FIRST PROGRAMING SESSION

You are now ready to enjoy a delightful few minutes of restful repose.

It can be the most valuable few minutes you have ever spent. Here are five steps to follow. Read first.

HOW TO: ENJOY A USEFUL PROGRAMING SESSION

1. Relax your body and mind. Use any of the three methods that appeal to you. Or, do all three together. First the Eye, then the Breathing, then the Head-to-Toe Technique.
2. See yourself at your proper weight. Refresh your memory with an album picture of yourself slender, if necessary.
3. Say to yourself, "I enjoy protein foods more and more every day. Foods that are good for my body taste good to me."
4. Say to yourself, "I will relax and program myself at least once a day, making each session easier and more effective day by day." See yourself doing it.
5. Say to yourself, "I am going to end my session at the count of three feeling wonderful, better than I felt before." Then count aloud or to yourself, "One, Two, THREE!"

Read these five steps over again. Review the relaxation techniques. Go one step at a time to become familiar with each, if you feel the five steps are too much to remember. Actually, all you do is relax, visualize, make two statements, then end your session.

Ready? Do it now.

PROGRAMING YOURSELF TO EAT PROPERLY
WITHOUT THE NEED FOR SACRIFICE, AIMLESS DISCIPLINE,
OR WILLPOWER

You now have three different techniques to induce a relaxed state, ready to accept mental programing.

Choose the one or two techniques that are natural and enjoyable for you.

There is just one method to end your session. All you do is count—"One, Two, THREE!"

Although your entire session may last only a few minutes, you will feel great afterwards. You will be rested, re-charged, and vitalized. A relaxed state is a very therapeutic state to experience. You will want to do it more than once a day.

But the gold nuggets on this path are the programings you give yourself before you count to three.

You could place these into four categories:

- Programing for proper eating generally.
- Programing to supplant specific problem foods or specific unwanted eating habits.
- Programing for wholesome, creative attitudes generally.
- Programing to supplant specific emotions or attitudes that ring appetite bells.

Let's first examine the simple ways to program yourself for proper eating.

We mentioned one way already—see yourself thin. Well, if you look at this in the light of the four programing categories, you see this fits all four. It is an umbrella type of programing that reinforces all the specific programing we will now spell out. It is, therefore, the most important programing of all.

Learn to see yourself as you want to be, vividly and realistically. An old photograph of yourself is usually helpful. When you program yourself with a slender image of you, be elated, be enthusiastic, be assured—know it will be so. And so it will become.

Now for the programing for proper eating.

Here is one of the most effective methods I know:

HOW TO: PROGRAMING FOR EFFORTLESS HIGH PROTEIN DINING

1. Make a list of high protein foods that you will include on your menus (beef, lamb, poultry, fish, eggs, etc.).
2. Make a list of the sweets and starches you will eliminate once and for all (baked goods, pastas, candy, cereals, etc.).
3. Perform your relaxation session with the list of non-fattening foods in your right hand and the list of fattening foods in your left hand.
4. Program yourself as follows: "I enjoy the high protein foods listed in

my right hand. These foods bring me satisfaction and nourish my body. I have no appetite or need for the foods on the high carbohydrate list in my left hand. I reject them."

5. Crumple the left hand list and throw it on the floor as you end your session: "I end my session on the count of three feeling great. One, Two, THREE."

Here is another good programing statement to help increase affirmation in your relaxation session:

"I have no need for empty calories in sweet and starchy foods. Thus I have no desire for high carbohydrate content or nutritionally depleted foods. Foods high in nutrition appeal to me. I enjoy high protein, high mineral, high vitamin foods."

And another, this one to ease up on quantity:

"High protein foods on my slenderizing program taste so delicious and are so satisfying that I require smaller portions and have very little need to eat between meals."

Understand the idea?
Use your own words.
Use your own pictures.
Keep the words positive and the pictures real.
In a few programing sessions, you will have to pinch yourself to believe you are actually eating correctly without effort or sacrifice.
And there will be less of you to pinch.

REPROGRAMING YOURSELF OUT OF PIZZA, DOUGHNUTS, CANDY OR OTHER STUBBORN FATTENING "FOODS"

Programing must be positive. It should emphasize what you are to do, not what you are not to do.

Negative programing often has a built-in canceling effect. For instance, suppose you had an irresistible penchant for fudge. If you were to program yourself, "I will no longer enjoy fudge," you are not giving yourself something to do, you are creating a vacuum by giving yourself something not to do, putting no substitute in its place.

The psychologists have what they call the Law of Reverse Effect. Tell a child to be careful and not spill his milk, but be prepared to drag out the mop.

The very mention of "don't spill" increases the likelihood of spilling because you cannot "not do" something. Programing is for action. There is no action in "not do."

The very mention of fudge in programing to "not enjoy" increases the likelihood of action involving fudge. And you know what action this suggests.

It is always desirable to program for positive action:

"Whenever I have the desire for fudge, I will have no-cal soda instead. It will be much more enjoyable than fudge. It will satisfy and dispel my craving."

This is the substitution method. It substitutes one food for another. There is positive action in this programing.

It is best to use positive, healthful suggestions. Use those described in the previous section of this chapter, or create your own. . . .

One warning. . . .

PROGRAMING SHOULD BE ELASTIC AND PERMISSIVE

Never give yourself iron-clad commands. Make the programing permissive in nature. "I enjoy the proper foods" is more desirable than "I eat only beef, lamb, poultry, fish, eggs."

Such definitive programing eliminates from your desire the natural fresh vegetables and fruits that are essential for your nutrition.

True, I want you to keep an eye on your intake of fruits and vegetables until you reach your desired weight. But a portion a day of salad or vegetable and fruit is a *must*.

As I said before, I am not in favor of the no fat or no carbohydrate diets that are now in vogue. I am *for* a high protein, low fat, low carbohydrate intake as detailed in Chapter 3.

I openly oppose an all protein diet and an all protein and fat diet. In this *no* carbohydrate approach, there are too many risks, including low blood sugar and excessive ketones or acid, in the system. There is also the possibility of breaking down essential tissue and the shortage of vital nutrients, etc.

Program yourself for eating properly, healthfully, without rigid, restrictive and unnatural requirements.

A tall, attractive girl, H.L., began taking Kung Fu to accelerate her mind control. She found she became "master of myself." Her motivation to lose weight increased. "I refuse to allow myself to become fat again." How much of her success was due to Kung Fu she found it hard to say. "All I know is—I am more relaxed, less shy with people, and my thoughts are less downgrading of myself, more positive. I walk briskly. My voice and eyes are brighter. I smile and laugh more. I am able to cope with problems in my life."

Kung Fu, or just plain you, it doesn't matter just so there is attention to the inner self. The outer package that affects the scale can then respond quickly and permanently.

PROGRAMING YOURSELF FOR PROPER ATTITUDES AND A POSITIVE, CONFIDENT SELF-IMAGE

As you know, eating properly is only one part of your program.

It is just as important to think about yourself, write about yourself, know yourself, love yourself. This is a unique part of my program, a part with which most physicians will agree.

If you look back, I have devoted six previous chapters to *you* and only one to food.

"You seem to care." I hear that so often from my patients. Some patients write letters of appreciation about how I have helped them to love themselves through self-understanding and reprograming.

Basically, what I have been telling you in these chapters about *you* is how to develop awareness of your own thoughts, feelings or emotions, attitudes and actions.

Be your own Siamese twin. Observe yourself.

Note your rationalizations and excuses. Write them down. Compare them to those in Chapter 2.

Develop awareness of what you say. Before you say it, while you are saying it, and after you say it. Also develop awareness of what you think, eat and do.

Remember to remember. Remember not to forget.

I give you this as part of your basic psychological programing.

HOW TO: PROGRAMING FOR SELF-AWARENESS

Relax. See yourself remembering to be aware of yourself. See yourself carrying pad and pen and writing about your favorite rationalizations or excuses. Say to yourself: "I am aware of my thoughts and why I think them. I am aware of my attitudes and why I have them. I am aware of my feelings and why I feel the way I do. I am aware of my actions and why I behave as I do. Every day I become more and more aware; therefore, every day in every way I become better and better and better."

Do it now.

As you develop more awareness about yourself you discern negative emotions. Pessimism, jealousy, fear, uncertainty, self-doubt, hatred, self-pity, vindictiveness, worry, anxiety. The list can be a long one. And if the true cause of death were to be listed on tombstones, there would be one or more such negative words on every grave.

Positive thinking is a life changer. Dr. Norman Vincent Peale's book,* "The Power of Positive Thinking" broke all best selling records. Millions of people have read it and turned their lives around from failure to success.

HOW TO: PROGRAMING FOR POSITIVE THINKING

Program yourself for positive thinking. Relax. See yourself enthusiastic and optimistic. The image you hold of yourself is a slender, happy, positive person as you say, "Positive thinking is my way of thinking. As I think and do positively, all the benefits I desire are mine."

Here is a Pavlov bell disconnector. If a negative feeling persists, this programing helps to disconnect it from your true hunger mechanism. You may continue to feel self-pity, for instance, but that self-pity won't continue to make you feel the urge to eat. Actually, your conscious mind will learn to understand this feeling and will not permit you to eat.

HOW TO: PROGRAMING FOR DISCONNECTING
EMOTION FROM APPETITE

Relax. See yourself paying attention to your emotions instead of burying them under a stack of pancakes or other food. Say to yourself,

---

*Prentice-Hall, Inc., Englewood Cliffs, N.J.

"Appetite is triggered by a new bell for me. It means I am starved for self-attention. Whenever I feel appetite without true stomach hunger, I will honor it with sincere self-study and attention toward better understanding and fulfilling my emotional needs."

HOW TO ZERO IN ON SPECIAL HANG-UPS THAT RING APPETITE BELLS, THEN SILENCE THEM

Suppose you are aware of yourself and find yourself saying, "It is becoming more difficult to lose weight."

You recognize this as a "cop out." You don't want that statement to program you. So what do you do about it?

Here is what you do.

HOW TO: PROGRAMING OUT COP-OUT AND DROP-OUT PHRASES

As soon as you spot yourself saying the unwanted phrase, relax immediately or as soon thereafter as possible and say to yourself, "That phrase is no longer needed by me. I file it away in the inactive storage file of my subconscious. Instead, I accept as my active programing, the statement ('Every day I am more at ease with myself and my weight is easier to control'—the positive counterpart of the unwanted statement.) This is a beautiful statement. I use it freely." When you end your session, write about the positive counterpart a few times on a piece of paper to become more familiar with it.

You can do the same with specific attitudes that you identify on your mental safaris as food-dangerous.

You can cancel out remorse and feel forgiveness. Or you can turn "down" periods into "up" periods.

When you have identified an event in your life to which you react negatively, thereby setting off a chain-eating reaction (as you learned to do in Chapters 4 through 7), here is how you can program out this event so it ceases to "bug" your appetite.

HOW TO: REPROGRAM PAST EVENTS FOR LITTLE TO NO EFFECT ON PRESENT EMOTIONS OR APPETITE

Relax. Say to yourself, "I no longer need to feel _____ (describe negative emotion). It is the result of _____ (describe negative event). This event is no longer of interest to me. Instead, I feel more and more _____ (describe positive counterpart of negative emotion) with every passing day."

OTHER VALUABLE PROGRAMING TO REACH YOUR GOAL

I think you are beginning to understand the idea.

By relaxing deeply, you open your subconscious computer or servo-mechanism for programing.

You visualize or affirm your new instructions. It becomes part of your natural habits almost immediately.

You repeat these programing sessions daily and you reinforce them.

You end negative attitudes. You develop new, positive attitudes. You end improper eating. You begin proper eating—naturally, effortlessly, and soon it will become routine the rest of your life.

There are no magic mental pictures. No abracadabra incantations.

All of the programing is down to earth common sense. You can formulate your own programing to fit your own attitudes and behavior patterns.

However, before I end this chapter and go on to other methods to obtain insight about yourself for reprograming, here are additional examples of food and emotion programing.

First, programing food and eating habits.

Here are a few ideas you may use in your own programing instructions and pictures:

"The more I eat, the more bloated and uncomfortable I feel. A modest meal leaves me satisfied and at a high level of well-being."

"I have no need, emotionally or bodily, for sweet and starchy foods. High protein foods give me both emotional and bodily satisfaction."

"I have no desire to eat candy. My desire is to eat nutritional foods. I have no desire for the fat that candy becomes." Here, of course, you can insert other troublesome carbohydrate foods.

"I picture myself gagging on foods heavy in sweets and starches. I picture myself eating happily and effortlessly the foods low in carbohydrates."

"I am able to enjoy a caffeine-free coffee break with no desire for deadening pastry or cake. The coffee break without carbohydrate accompaniment is much more rejuvenating and uplifting for me."

"My regular meals are all I need. Additional food between meals adds only unwanted fat. I enjoy my regular meals much more when I refrain from eating between meals."

Next, programing for a healthier frame of mind (emotions).

"I see the best in other people and in myself. What is less than good is still undeveloped and not ready to be seen. I see people and myself as flowers unfolding."

"Despite all adversity, I know progress is being made. I concentrate less on the problems of life and more on the solutions."

"I do not keep my hurt feelings a secret. I air them, share them and thus repair them."

"I am not afraid to love others or myself. I know I receive only as much love as I give. So I give freely."

"My relaxation sessions program me for greater sexual pleasure by releasing tensions and dispelling frustrations. I enjoy sexual relations more and more."

"I am an effective person. I have a combination of strong points and personal assets possessed by no one else. I am confident. I am successful. Whatever goal I set, I reach."

Meat of Chapter 8

The meat of the program is programing. Learn how to induce relaxation by the several techniques shown, then give yourself the images or verbal affirmations that you need to:

1. Program yourself for proper, high protein eating.
2. Program yourself for positive, high-spirited living.

Do several relaxation sessions with one or two devoted to food, one or two devoted to emotions and attitudes, etc.

Before you end each session on the count of three, see yourself enjoying these programing sessions daily, feeling more deeply relaxed each time, and more capable of developing the best slenderizing program.

9

THE AMAZING REDUCING POWER
OF A POSITIVE SELF-IMAGE

Appetizer for Chapter 9

Did you ever go to a carnival and look into those crazy mirrors? Some make you unbelievably tall, some hilariously short and fat. Well, have I got a mirror for you!

A man has ulcers. He is a constant worrier and now the negativity is taking its toll. He goes to the hospital. He starts a bland diet—the whole treatment. He recovers and returns to the office.

It's the same office with the same problems. And it is the same man. Man + worry = ulcers. Naturally, in a few months, the ulcers return. This time his doctor warns him upon leaving the hospital, he should go on an extended trip or take a long, restful vacation.

He does. When he returns he is feeling fine, rarin' to jump into harness again. But he is still the same man and it is still the same office. You know the end to the story. Back and forth to the hospital until something changes—the man or the office.

Do you see the corollary with the overweight person? The diet to cure the ill. The return of the weight. There can be no cure, no permanent slenderness, until either the person or the environment changes.

It is often not possible to change your environment. A family is a family. One cannot always pull up stakes.

So it is the person who must change.

Some people leave the program because they run into life's problems too early—before they learn how to handle them without resort to their alimentary canal. One woman found that her 14-year old daughter was pregnant. She guided her through the distress, the abortion, the aftermath without losing her stride in the program. Had it happened earlier—before she began to realize the connection between problems and portions—she could easily have lost months of progress.

On the other hand J.H., a divorcee who had recently remarried, couldn't cope with her new husband's alcoholism. She left the program and re-entered several times. Then came the insight. She reached her goal and brought her husband in for help.

For some people oral satisfaction is so important they refuse to understand many things, including their inner emotional nature. So they continue eating and drop out of the program. Fortunately, they are the exceptions.

R.K., age 17, was not motivated more than ten weeks. She dropped 25 pounds, then gained back five and quit.

B.L. quit in two months after losing three pounds and gaining back four. He never wrote a word.

A.W. quit in one month. He expected me to do all the work. So his weight also went up instead of down.

You can't be a winner all the time.

For you to stop pounding that treadmill, pound after stupid pound, you have to change.

I am not talking about changing your desire, your positiveness, your perseverance, your determination. Lord knows you've revved those up to full throttle many times in the past. It doesn't work.

I'm talking about you, dear reader, the inner, the real, the living *you*. And *you* know exactly who I mean.

THE IMAGE YOU HOLD OF YOURSELF IS A BLUEPRINT FOR THE BODY

"Yes," you say, "I know who you mean, but how can I change *me*?"

Chapter 8 gave you the method. Now, in this chapter, you shall learn a powerful way to apply this method.

I have hinted at it before. I have asked you to program yourself for weight and fat loss by visualizing yourself slim.

Some of you must have read this and figured I was smoking something or losing my marbles. Sometimes seeing yourself thin is merely wishful thinking, a lazy person's way of dreaming about something he hasn't the guts to attain.

You are lying on the living room couch with the television on and a box of candy within finger reach and you see a lovely female on the screen. You dream about being as slender as she is or slender enough to attract her if you are a male. This is not programing. It is wishful dreaming.

But if you are sitting in a straight back chair using a relaxation technique and you picture yourself becoming as slender as you desire, you are programing yourself. You may be dreaming a dream but there's a difference. This dream is coming true.

What is the real difference? In the television case, you are in touch with a box of chocolate. In the latter case, you are in touch with your subconscious. You are holding an image of you in your mind that is different than you are now. You are in effect changing your self-image. Now here's the important part:

Your self-image is the blueprint of *you*. When you change the blueprint of anything, you change the product, whether it is a machine, a built-in, a lamp or a house.

Certainly, the expression of our consciousness through our body is evident in sickness and in health. A consciousness of worry produces ulcers. A consciousness of strain and anxiety affects the heart. The psychosomatic aspects of most illnesses are being more readily recognized and understood by the medical profession.

A man who helps to program electronic computers is called a computer programer. A man who helps to program people is called a hypnologist.

Patients frequently consult hypnotists for reprograming in order to correct a number of physical conditions. These include ailments you may think are totally unrelated to the person's consciousness, state of mind, or self-image, such as—gastrointestinal disorders, respiratory problems, heart conditions, skin problems, etc.

Chronic ulcerative colitis is known to be caused by severe psychic strain. Hypnotic reconditioning or reprograming can relieve this strain and produce a corresponding improvement in the condition.

The power of the mind over the body is seemingly miraculous. The rules say one thing, but if the mind says another, the body obeys the mind.

Is there any wonder why a person continues to manifest an overweight body as long as he is used to seeing himself as an overweight person?

You have to change your mind to change your weight.

HOW TO CUSTOM BUILD A MENTAL IMAGE
THAT WILL CREATE A NEW PHYSICAL BODY

Do you mind standing for a moment and bringing your book over to the largest mirror in the house, preferably a full length mirror? You may return in a few minutes . . .

Now take a long look at yourself. See room for improvement? How? List three top priority areas you desire to change in your mirror image. One of these will no doubt be a more slender profile but be more specific.

- Five inches off the hips
- Two inches off the neck
- Two inches off each thigh
- Three inches off the bust or chest
- Four inches off the waist

You may also see other areas for improvement, such as:

- Straighter posture
- Clearer complexion
- Neater appearance
- Better coiffure
- Happier look

There are possibly other areas of improvement that don't meet everyone's eye. But when you see yourself in the mirror, you see the inner self, too. How about listing a few areas of improvement there:

- More self-confidence
- Able to eat properly

- Derives more satisfaction from people
- Sees the sunny side of life
- Makes everything that happens happen for the best

You do not have to choose from the five physical measurements, the five aspects of appearance, or the five behavioral aspects I have listed. There are certainly scores of others which could be listed, but I don't want to create a new picture of *you*. I want *you* to do it. I want you to be the creator of your new body, your new personality, your new and happier circumstances in life.

What does the new image of you reflect? List three top priority changes in

Physical Measurements
Appearance
Behavior

Now stand in front of the mirror again and see these changes occurring before your very eyes. See the physical measurements improve. See your appearance improve in three ways. See yourself behaving and feeling as you have now specified.

> D.J. was a tall, "shocking" redhead. At 6'4" most of her excess pounds (she weighed 161) were on her legs and rear end. "She appeared to be a witch when she came in," recalls my nurse. "Too much black make-up on her eyes and a very loud voice."
>
> Two months later, D.J. had learned much about herself, thinking and writing. She had done some reprograming. Now she was 17 pounds lighter, a more slender figure, wore less make-up and perfume, also her voice and manner were toned down and feminine.

Have a good, long look at these imagined changes in you. They are not yet real in the mirror. But allow a dreamy over-image superimpose itself between your eyes and the mirror image.

This is your new custom-built self-image.

It is the blueprint of things to come.

Do you let it go at that?

Not on your life.

You now go back to your chair, set the book down, and . . .

HOW TO: PROGRAM YOURSELF FOR YOUR NEW SELF-IMAGE

Relax very deeply.
See yourself with all these new attributes.
End your session with positive programing.

RX FOR AN IMAGE OF A SUCCESSFUL YOU

You have tried to be slender and have failed.

You have tried again and again to abstain from eating fattening foods, but again and again have put them in your mouth.

You have made resolution after resolution, then broken resolution after resolution.

Each of these failures—and there have been countless, right?—have programed you for continued failure.

Listen to some of my patients talk about their failures. Can you visualize their negative programing?

"I didn't do too well since I was last in the office. I still crave sweets." (*Coming up.* One large helping of failure.)

"I had my weight under control once. I know there's no reason I can't again. If only for my husband's sake." (Note the negative approach, "no reason," "can't" instead of "every reason," "can," and get the safety ejection seat ready to go—one wrong move by her husband.)

"I know what my problems are but I don't seem to want to do anything about it. I stick to it for awhile, then seem to go off. I always seem to go back to the same old habits." (Is there any better way of saying "I am programed to be the way I am; every effort to be otherwise will fail.")

"My weight is coming off slowly. It's like pulling teeth." (How long can pulling teeth last? Even if you're a horse.)

"I get so mean one week before my period. I even get mean to myself and overeat." (Age 34, she'll be having her periods for a long time—and her excuse for failure.)

These patients need to reprogram themselves for success.

They can use the relaxation method, but there's a hitch. Remember, you must expect success when you use this method. And it works only to the extent that you expect and cooperate (think and do).

Now, if you are programed for failure, this becomes a very insidious thing. It can undermine all other programing.

"It won't work."
"I've tried that."
"My friend tried it. It didn't do anything for her."
"That's ridiculous."
"I can't relax."
"I can't picture myself thin."
"I'll do it, but we'll see . . ."

Wilson Mizner said once, "The gent who wakes up and finds himself a success hasn't been asleep." People who are programed for failure have in all likelihood been unaware of what they were thinking and doing. They have been asleep, at least concerning the failure habit they have been reinforcing for several years.

But you are awake. You are aware. You know now what you have been doing. You realize that appetite bells ring and the appetite is false. You realize that mouth hunger can pretend to be stomach hunger. You know yourself more intimately. You see how, in the past, you have reinforced failure patterns instead of rejecting them in favor of success patterns.

As long as you are awake in the sense that *you are aware,* you are in control. You can turn your failure expectation into success expectation merely by understanding the past, closing the door on it, and expecting a new, success-packed future.

People who have seen the true nature of their failure patterns as conditioning for failure, programing for failure, have been able to do something about it.

- Shy people have become outgoing.
- Timid speakers have become public orators.
- Job holders have risen the ladder to executive posts.
- Jittery people have become virtually unshakeable.
- Poor golfers have become golf champions.
- Smokers have found it easy to undo the habit.

And, of course, overweight people have found it easy to change the overeating and improper eating habit.

I promise you things will change in your life when you begin thinking about yourself as very important in this program.

S.V., 50, dropped out of the program. She found it was too much effort to discipline her palate. "Not if you allow time to think," I urged, to no avail.

She returned after awhile when one of her friends related the amazing results which occur when you think about yourself.

She thought. And as she thought, it became easier. Her weight sank 20 pounds in two months. Here's how she describes some other changes:

> "I feel so wonderful. I've discovered myself. I have a better attitude. I'm not bothered and upset as easily with my husband the way I used to be.
>
> "I can slip into a size 9 dress and look good. I used to overeat when depressed. Now I don't eat all the time and make a hog of myself. I know it's unnecessary now and I have this in my head.
>
> "I have dresses that I couldn't wear before—size 5—and they almost fit me now. I was wearing a size 12 and 14 before. I want to dress and do things.
>
> "I have a new puppy and enjoy taking him for a walk. Another thing, I used to have hot flashes constantly at night. Now, no more hot flashes and I sleep the night through just like a new born baby.
>
> "No more aches and pains in my legs. I can awaken early and do all my housework in a few hours. No backaches. I have a lot of energy and desire to do other things—reading, knitting, making decal pictures, candles (for our club bazaar and Christmas time), bike riding. I never did this before."

There are many cases where patience, thought, persistence and well-directed effort help shape a new self-image—a MIRACLE.

How have you programed yourself for failure? Are these some of your rationalizations (excuses)?

> "I have decided to start on a diet, then put it off again and again."
>
> "I have started on a diet, then ended it before I actually went anywhere with it."
>
> "I have dieted and lost, then slipped back into my old habits and regained."
>
> "I have been on a diet and eaten taboo things time and time again."
>
> "My overweight condition means that I fail to attract the person I admire."
>
> "My overweight interferes with the work I do."
>
> "My overweight loses me friends, jobs and opportunities."

Failure, failure, failure.

Let's turn it around right now.

HOW TO: PROGRAM OUT FAILURE, PROGRAM IN SUCCESS

Relax very deeply. Repeat to yourself, "I am not a failure. I am a success person. I know this to be true now. I am able to do anything I desire. My capability for success is as great, if not greater than other people I know. I see myself concentrating more and more on my accomplishments as my success pattern is permitted to unfold and enlarge."

You must now reinforce this programing by patting yourself on the back whenever you do well. Feel no remorse about the occasional slips. Let them slip away.

Dwell on your successes.

HOW TO KEEP SUCCESS FIRMLY IMPLANTED

Weight loss is a great deceiver.

You weigh yourself. You weigh less. Yet you may have merely dehydrated yourself.

You weigh yourself. You weigh more. Yet you may have actually shed some fat.

If you think "weight *loss*," you may be paving the way to find again whatever you have lost.

Pay less attention to hour-to-hour or day-to-day weight. Don't be obsessed with weight loss per se. Instead, become involved in your weight *program*.

When you play the "pound" game, you permit yourself to win or lose.

When you play the "time" game, you invite success or failure.

Don't invite the possibility of failure by setting such meaningless goals. Let there be room only for success—a successful weight control program.

Another trap is pitting you against yourself. If there is to be such a contest, one of you surely will fail. Failure must be blocked out. You are not supposed to be battling yourself, you are spending time with yourself. You are learning to understand yourself. There can be no losers now.

Reinforce your pattern for successful progress by reviewing all the correct programing you did during the day. Make this a regular ritual before you retire at night. Review the proper foods you ate, the times you didn't eat when in the past you may have. Review all the moments of self-awareness, how you thought about yourself, wrote about yourself, received insight about yourself.

Feel good about these good things. Give yourself a mental pat on the back. Know that tomorrow will be successful.

This is no idle talk. You can, I'm sure, understand what you are doing when you review success before falling asleep at night.

You are relaxed. So your subconscious mind is prime for programing.

Were you to visualize the cake you ate and were you to feel guilty, you would be programing a self-image of food failure. If you're pushing mental buttons that program an image of you as a weak-willed glutton, you're setting yourself up for that kind of a tomorrow.

Instead, think about what you did right. You feel good about it. Now you are programing yourself for even greater successes tomorrow.

"Have you been thinking properly?" I asked a local business man who came to see me for the third time. He had lost about fifteen pounds, which was fine, but I had expected more of him—to go down the drain.

"Yes, whenever I have the chance, I spend time with myself," he said.

"Don't leave it to chance," I offered. He understood, and weighs much less today.

The weight takes care of itself when you take care of yourself. Take care of yourself by thinking and programing yourself more in the successful ways we have discussed.

For you to have fun on this program, you must make it as easy as possible. Believe me, it's possible to make it extremely easy. The easier, the more successful you are with the program each day.

And success breeds success.

THE SCALE AS A MEASURE OF SUCCESS

We have a running discussion among bariatric physicians which seems to pop up regularly. We evaluate our success, so our colleagues can judge the efficiency of our methods. This evaluation is often based on the average pounds lost per patient, or on what percent of our patients lost 20 pounds, or 40 pounds.

Now this has many faults. Some physicians don't count patients who do not return a second time, or who drop out from treatment somewhere along the way. What good is a treatment method that boasts 100 percent success when only 25 percent of the patients *stick* long enough to be counted?

As to pounds lost, 20 pounds is a satisfactory loss for a 140-pound woman, but is it a successful loss for a 280-pound man?

We are still searching for a fair way to weigh success.

Should you weigh your success only on the scale?

I say there are many faults in using the scale as the sole measure of your success.

Suppose you weigh five pounds less, but are miserable, tense, and having a real hard time. That is not progress.

On the other hand if you weigh only two pounds less, but are happier, more at ease, full of energy and enthusiasm, that is progress.

Remember, when you create your self-image of success, don't put the scale in the picture unless it adds to the success picture. You can make successful progress in the program by:

- Losing inches
- Learning to know yourself
- Turning off false appetites
- Becoming more positive
- Acquiring calm and tranquility
- Improving your health
- Improving your body tone and skin radiance

If you are successful in at least one of these areas, you have reason to see yourself in a success pattern. More will follow. Yes, even the scale.

I wonder whether, with Women's Lib, there will be more overweight men. When men are not home, women worry what they are up to, and they eat, munch and snack away the time. If women had as much freedom, the stay-at-home men could be the ones to eat-to-relieve-the-suspicion.

One women's husband was a musician who worked late every

night. He would bring her snacks, such as fried clams, hamburgers, French fries at 2:00 a.m. He knew she would become suspicious of him if she lost interest in eating and snacking.

I remember that she bought a pig for her charm bracelet the day she started on the program at 245 pounds. It was engraved with her goal of 150.

Soon she was refusing her husband's late snacks and making him answer for his late wanderings. It was too late to save the marriage ("I'm glad he's gone, I can fall asleep before midnight."). She found a job as a telephone operator and reached her goal in 4½ months, happy, years younger in appearance, and an emotionally stable woman.

THE WEIGHT-REDUCING EFFECTS OF AN
ACTIVE SELF-IMAGE

So much for the success factor in the image you have of yourself. I have discussed it in more detail because, next to the image of yourself slender, the image of yourself successful at whatever you do is vital.

There are other important ingredients of this self-image.

U.S. Surgeon General Jesse Steinfeld was recently quoted as observing that "The only exercise some people do is jumping to conclusions, sidestepping responsibilities, and pushing their luck."

Obviously, he is talking about overweight people. Are overweight people sluggish in their activity because of those extra pounds they must carry? Or, are overweight people overweight because they are sluggish in their activity?

I don't know which came first, the chicken or the egg, but I do know obesity and exercise are incompatible. If you are content to be overweight, you don't enjoy exercising. If you do exercise, you chase away excess pounds.

This is not an exercise book. You already know how to exercise. Some people consider calisthenics an exercise in futility. I know there are many good physical benefits from exercise. If you are an active person, you are exercising productively, and helping your body shed unwanted pounds.

Now here's a bonus you never thought you would receive with this book: Do you know you can relax, visualize yourself active and gain many of the physical benefits from such mental exercises?

It's true. Professional golfers often practice for a tournament on a new golf course by sitting in an arm chair and mentally playing the course in a few minutes. They actually become more familiar with the course and how to play it. Certainly, they have to play the course at least once. Then, by mental images, they can "play" 72 holes in a pouring rain in less than an hour.

If you sit in your chair and picture yourself playing nine holes of golf, you won't expend 2,000 extra calories or lose half a pound, but the programing for golf or just plain accelerated activity does have an effect.

HOW TO: ADD ACTIVITY TO YOUR SELF-IMAGE

See yourself physically active.
See yourself moving faster.
See yourself doing some sitting up exercises.
See yourself walking instead of riding.
See yourself climbing a few flights instead of riding the elevator.

Visualizing yourself active while sitting in a quiet state of programability mentally conditions you into a more active life.
Here is how it works:

1. Seeing yourself active gives you a self-image of being an active person.
2. The self-image being the blueprint of you, you find it more natural to be active.
3. Doing what comes naturally requires less effort, so being a more active person becomes almost effortless for you.
4. Since it now requires less effort to be active, you move faster, walk more, do more.
5. You burn more calories and become the slender self you should and can be.

HOW TO COMPLETE THE SPECIFICATIONS FOR YOUR NEW SELF-IMAGE

It requires only a few minutes a day to create a new self-image, paving the way for a great, new life.

One woman who programed herself for a new self-image every

morning on arising told me it required only three minutes a morning and only five mornings—a total of 15 minutes. "I'm beginning to feel something good is finally happening to me," she reported. It was. She lost 45 pounds within five months. It may require more or less time depending on how well you are able to relax and visualize; also, depending on how vast a change you need to make in your self-image.

Is it worth 15 minutes, more or less? You can bet your life it is.

In this chapter so far we have discussed six ways to improve your self-image:

1. A general picture of yourself thin.
2. A mirror picture of inches off.
3. A mirror picture of better posture, etc.
4. A mirror picture of proper eating and positive emotional behavior.
5. The quality of success.
6. The quality of activity.

These are priority specifications for your new self-image. The order depicted above is rather meaningful, too.

You begin with a general view of yourself thin as you would wish to be, enjoying life as a slender person. Then, focus sharper on that picture (2, 3, and 4). Next, convert your self-image from one of failure to success. You are then ready to "get a move on" in step 6.

This is not the whole self-image picture. Many of the programing steps I described in Chapter 8 have to do with your self-image.

For example, health. If you're on this program, you are going to feel healthy. If you persist in seeing yourself as a person that is chronically ill or in pain, you're programing yourself for sickness, not health.

On the other hand, if you make radiant, good health a part of your self-image—and program yourself for this self-image daily— you can hasten the day when your aches and pains go the way of all excess flesh.

I know overweight women who were plagued with heavy menstrual flow. Part of their slender self-image included a picture of themselves free of this problem. When they approached this slender image, the menstrual part of their mental picture corrected itself, too.

Overweight men and women are favorite targets for diabetes, high blood pressure and many other diseases. If you are such a target, visualize yourself free of the health problem in your self-image programing.

Complete the specifications for your new self-image in all the physical and psychological ways you can recall.

See yourself perfect inside and out.

"I LOOK IN THE MIRROR AND THERE'S NO ONE THERE"

I keep referring to your self-image. I assume you know what I mean. Most of you do. Yet there are some people who cannot subjectively "see" themselves. They actually don't know how they appear to others.

If you try to visualize your spouse or a parent right now, you may find it difficult. A person with whom we have close and frequent contact often presents a hazy visual image. The image has given way to a vague concept.

You may see yourself in the mirror and are so accustomed to seeing yourself you cannot depreciate or appreciate who and what you see.

For those who have this difficulty, I am going to hand you a different mirror to gaze into—a total concept mirror.

It is actually not a mirror. It is a personality profile in the form of a questionnaire. Still, it reflects *you*.

You can jot down your answers in less than a minute. Then you can program yourself for changes where they seem warranted.

Do this form now. First, write the letters A, B, C, D, E, F, G, H, I, and J in a column down the left side of a piece of paper. Opposite each letter, write the numbers 1, 2, 3, 4.

PERSONALITY PROFILE FOR AID IN CORRECTIVE PROGRAMING

(Read each group of statements in a category. Using pen and paper, note the statements best describing the way you think and feel now.)

Category A. Weight

1. I feel thoroughly discouraged about my overweight problem.
2. I feel somewhat dejected about weighing too much.
3. I feel hopeful about ending my weight problem.
4. I feel enthusiastic about this program and see myself slenderizing on it.

Category B. Success

1. I see myself as a complete failure in just about everything I do.
2. I fail more often than I succeed.
3. I fail occasionally.
4. I am successful with most things I undertake.

Category C. Self-Appreciation

1. I can't stand myself.
2. I am occasionally disgusted with myself.
3. I disappoint myself at times, but am proud of myself at other times.
4. I have confidence in myself.

Category D. Appearance

1. I think of myself as ugly.
2. I am an unattractive person.
3. I'm not bad to look at.
4. I have basically attractive features.

Category E. Enjoyment

1. Nothing ever pleases me any more.
2. I don't have as much fun out of life as I once had.
3. I have no complaints.
4. I enjoy life.

Category F. Energy

1. I never have enough energy to do anything.
2. I tire easily.
3. I have enough energy to do many things.
4. I have more than enough energy to do whatever I desire.

Category G. Sociability

1. I keep to myself and have no interest in being with other people.
2. I prefer my own company to others.
3. I am equally comfortable alone or with other people.
4. I prefer to be with others than by myself.

Category H. Mood

1. I have no hope in the future.

2. I have little to which I look forward.

3. Tomorrow could be better or worse than today.

4. I am optimistic about the future.

Category I. Health

1. I am miserable most of the time.

2. First it's one thing then another.

3. I don't feel as well as I should.

4. I have no complaints. I feel good.

Category J. Purpose

1. I cannot make any decisions.

2. I procrastinate when it comes to setting a goal or making a decision.

3. I am ambitious but cannot seem to reach all my goals.

4. I set goals, make decisions and carry them out.

There is no need to add your score as it is not a test. It is unimportant whether your score is 30 or 35. What is important is the categories that indicate less than a score of 4.

Where you have scored less than 4, you definitely need programing to strengthen your opinion of yourself in that department.

Note I did not say "strengthen yourself in that department." I said "strengthen your opinion of yourself." This is an important difference.

Were you to sit down and program yourself for more energy, for instance, saying, "I have enough energy to do anything," when you just finished checking off "I never have energy to do anything," how much expectation and belief do you think you will be mustering? Not much.

However, it is easy to understand that you could become an energetic person once you *see* yourself as an energetic person. No limit on expectation and belief here. Result: successful programing.

Begin with the category where you scored the least. Use several programing sessions to restore your self-image in this category. Then go to work on others where you scored less than 4.

HOW TO: CORRECTIVE SELF-IMAGE PROGRAMING FOR PERSONALITY PROFILE CATEGORIES

Relax very deeply using your favorite technique. Then use this programing for each category needing reinforcement.

Category A. Weight
"I see myself at my proper weight. This is the real me. I am becoming myself."

Category B. Success
"I have an unlimited potential for success. I am able to realize that potential more and more every day."

Category C. Self-appreciation
"I see myself as a unique and able person. I have complete confidence in my capacity to solve problems and accomplish goals."

Category D. Appearance
"I see myself radiating *both* inner and outer beauty and attractiveness."

Category E. Enjoyment
"I see myself as a fun loving person, able to enjoy life and give enjoyment to others."

Category F. Energy
"I see myself as an energetic person always endowed with enough energy to do whatever I desire or must do."

Category G. Sociability
"I picture myself enjoying and being enjoyed by others."

Category H. Mood
"I picture myself as seeing the good side of problems and situations. I am optimistic and know that I can make everything happen for the best."

Category I. Health
"I can see myself radiantly healthy. I know that every day my health is improving."

Category J. Purpose
"I see myself as an effective person. I set goals, make decisions and carry them out. My present goal is to continue daily on my proper eating program. I see myself fitting into such a program effortlessly."

Let the focus of your self-image become sharper every time you program yourself.

Sure you have defects. You admit to them. You know more about them today than you did yesterday. And you will know yourself much better tomorrow.

Defects, like extra baggage, extra clothing, or extra weight, can be eliminated. You visualize yourself without these extras. You see yourself free of these unwanted defects, free of excess pounds.

You see yourself as you are meant to be.
And so you become.

Meat of Chapter 9

As you see yourself, so you become. You can custom build a new you. Begin with the blueprint—the image you have of yourself as you know you can be.

Beginning with physical measurements and going on to physical appearance and temperament or personality, you can create a clear and total picture of yourself. Accept that picture, then program it into your subconscious mind to replace the picture you previously had.

Do the programing session that fits you with new attributes. Make success an integral part of your self-image. Add other measures for success, such as inches instead of pounds, and learning to understand yourself. If you need to sharpen your self-image, use the Personality Profile Form. Program yourself wherever you need reinforcement so as to perfect this blueprint.

10

SECRET CONFESSIONS

OF OVERWEIGHT MEN

AND WOMEN AND HOW

THE ACT OF "CONFESSING"

HELPS YOU GROW THIN

Appetizer for Chapter 10

What are you having for breakfast this morning? Half a cantaloupe, three fried eggs, decaffeinated coffee? Great. And lunch? Hamburger steak with mushrooms and watercress? Perfect. What's for dinner? Onion soup, baked Chicken Tarragon, Brussels sprouts, and gelatine dessert? Wish I could be there. Hearty appetite! Not the false, emotional, reaction appetite. The real kind—hunger. In order to understand the difference, this chapter takes you inside the hearts of a number of people before and after they discovered there was a difference.

"I am afraid of marriage or a serious relationship. I don't want to make a mistake such as my parents did. When I go into a shell of fear, I eat . . . I really want to find myself, rid myself of fears, shells, habits, and be a free person."

Can you read the memories behind tne words? Can you imagine what lies inside the layers of blubber of this 180 pound, 27-year old woman. She could instead be writing . . .

"He's drunk again. Oh, God, he's hitting her. DON'T, DAD, DON'T!!"

Thoughts that flip in and out, such as "I don't want to make a mistake like my parents did" can escape our conscious mind so readily. Yet, these can be the very thoughts that unlock the secret behind our need to eat excessively or improperly.

When I ask my patients to write, I remind them they don't have to think about form. It doesn't have to be in story book style or similar to a letter or diary.

The important thing is that you write. Let it happen spontaneously. Develop the habit of writing, then whenever the urge hits you, there are writing materials available to write about yourself.

Then write naturally, as though you were talking to someone. Allow your thoughts to flow uninterrupted, unaffected by time or sequence or orderly progression.

HOW SOME OVERWEIGHT PEOPLE HAVE TRACED THE ORIGINS OF THEIR PROBLEM

"I never had a childhood. I raised my parents. Dad was outgoing, the life of the party. Mother suffered quietly. The martyr. They stayed together for my benefit. Then divorce. Today I'm schizophrenic according to my psychiatrist. He has ordered no more shows or public appearances, no dancing—my other personality. So I think more about my youth and feel sorry for myself.

"One of my first recollections of childhood is Dad coming home drunk with lipstick on him. Mom beat him over the head with a shoe. That didn't do any good. It happened again and again. So she began to take her hostility and rage out on me. I became the butt of her disappointment. I'm in my third year of treatment. I don't flip out anymore. That's how I became schizo—couldn't make a choice between either parent. As a schizo I wasn't serious about weight loss. Maybe I'm improving. Because I'm serious now."

This 27-year-old young lady weighed 159 when I saw her the first time. She was nervous and looked older than her years. In this instance psychiatric care helped her to realize her problem. It certainly made it easier for me to make her understand those thirty odd pounds of unwanted padding. When I last saw her a few months later, she was poised, youthful looking—and slender.

Not all problems are that fracturing to the personality. In fact, if not for extra weight, many would not believe there was a problem at all. Even with the extra weight, many feel the problem is with food, nothing deeper. Until they think—and write:

"It seems I was fat even as a baby. I look at my baby pictures and think that it wasn't fair I was born with rolls in my legs (which I still have).

"I always blamed it on heredity. All my relatives have heavy legs; therefore, I have heavy legs. And as I grew up nothing changed. I never remember it being a problem in childhood. I don't recall but I'm sure it was. The earliest I remember is junior high. All the girls were wearing knee socks but the guys told me not to. I looked better in socks rolled down to the ankles because knee socks made me look fatter. No one actually said so, but I knew. I never looked good in shorts, and gym class was always a problem.

"I learned modern dance in the 7th grade because in gym you had to play outside in front of the guys. Also in dance, we had a running test once a year which I used to dread. We would run on the boys' track, my thighs would be flapping and I would be panting.

"Strangely enough, I had a great social life and was quite popular. I held important positions in school and dated quite heavily. But I was always somewhat self-conscious.

"At that time the beach was quite a hangout and I was constantly making excuses to stay away. I didn't want anyone to see me in a bathing suit.

"It's not that I didn't try to lose weight. I had a couple of serious boyfriends even at that age whom I'm sure would have wanted me to be slimmer. They were always pinching bits of fat or asking why I didn't wear shorter skirts. It seemed hopeless though. No matter what you did, you ate. And if you didn't eat, people would think you were dieting, and that was horrible."

So it went until today. But writing about it today bore special meaning for her. "I recalled painful details of my youth," she told me. "I realize I can never be happy as an adult until I am satisfied with my appearance."

Motivation. Goal. Reprograming. Expectation. Results!

"What did you have for dinner last night?" I posed the question to a 59-year old hairdresser.

"Leg of lamb," she replied, "I had some friends over to dinner. They raved about it."

My next question would have been, "What else did you have?" But I was delighted. I had already discovered something much more important. You will also understand after you read what she had written about herself only a few months before:

"Fat is a crazy, little cocoon which shields me from many unwanted attentions. It turns off most men and endears me to many women. They love to find someone fatter than they are.

"That wasn't enough. Around that I built another cocoon. This is in the form of a business building and small apartment. Within these walls I am able to live and work alone.

"The exterior is kept in muted colors and there are no signs to indicate that a business exists here. Exist is a good word because that is what I barely do. At every opportunity I close completely and go to bed. I rarely accept a new patron and only because a few of them die each year.

"My cocoons are a put-off. I have other put-offs:

1. Impatience—especially with phone calls. I hang up quickly.

2. No time—always work odd hours so my free time will not coincide with the free time that others have.

3. No money—never make more than enough for current expenses. Refuse to raise prices.

4. Can't cook—don't want to learn.

5. No comforts—no rugs, no curtains, no extra beds or bedding, no table, few chairs which are always loaded down with books, pottery, odds and ends.

6. No clothes—when I say 'I have nothing to wear,' it really means 'I don't want to go.' At a very early age I can remember crying when my mother put a new dress on me. Also cried when I had to go to the movies.

7. Uniform—the very word means 'one form.' I feel that uniform makes me just a part of the background.

8. Books—I always carry one when I'm in waiting rooms or buses. People seldom persist in conversation when you're reading.

9. Fatigue—'Too tired' is always a good reason to squirm out of unwanted invitations."

"Besides put-offs, I also have cover-ups:

1. Darkness—I love it. Frequently stay awake all night because I love the feeling of being awake when others are sleeping.

2. Rain—love to be out in it. You can hardly see through it and everyone looks alike.

3. Fog—love the dampness of it and the closed-in feeling it gives me."

Now do you see what I was elated about? Here was a woman that had created a prison for herself. It was a prison with no rewards or privileges, except food. So she ate and ate.

When I first saw her she weighed a little over 200 pounds. I handled her with kid gloves for fear she would flee to her cocoon and not return. Indeed, this happened several times during the first year. After losing a few pounds she became interested in writing about herself.

Writing was safe. She could do it alone. Little did she realize the power of her pen was knocking down those prison walls.

During the first year she lost a little. Eventually she began writing and the weight loss accelerated. She was averaging five pounds a month and weighed 142 that final visit—when she was having friends over for dinner.

What that leg of lamb really said was, "Free at last. Free at last."

HOW TO PROBE YOUR MEMORY TODAY FOR YESTERYEARS' APPETITE DISTORTERS AND DISSOLVE THEM TOMORROW

You need not wait a year to break out of your prison of oppressive weight.

You can probe your subconscious in your straight back chair—the same chair you use for your relaxation and reprograming sessions.

First, you establish a "yes" and "no" finger signal system. It is a means of communication between you and your subconscious mind, where all past experiences are stored.

You place your hands on your lap.

You relax.

You instruct "yourself" that a raising up of the right index finger indicates "yes" and left index finger "no."

You test yourself by asking, "Is my name George Washington?" Since your name is not George Washington (if it is, my pardon, sir), your left index finger should rise involuntarily.

Next, you ask, "Is my name _____?" (Use your true name.) Now your right index finger should rise.

At first you may notice only an imperceptible movement in your finger. This can be increased by repeating the initial step of instructing "yourself" which finger will rise for "yes" and which for "no." Expect more and more pronounced finger movements.

Once you have established this code system, you are ready to probe your deepest memories for false appetite triggers.

First, you may want to uncover how far back they stem. This you can do by asking, "Whatever emotional factor or experience is causing my overeating, did it begin before I was 10 years old?"

If the answer is "no," you increase the age by five or ten year stages until you arrive at the correct age bracket. Then by additional questions you can narrow it down to the very year.

Once you have the time established, you need to pinpoint the place, the people, the type of incident, and finally the exact incident.

The more you discover, the more you will know what line of questioning to use. It may require only twenty or thirty questions to discover that your propensity for second and third helpings or extra meals stem from Grandma's insistence, or the time the family ran out of money, or your return from the armed services.

Then write all about it. Capture this information for further thought, further writing about yourself, further understanding.

Understanding opens up the dam and permits the flood of fat to flow away.

Do it now.

HOW TO: PROBE THE SUBCONSCIOUS FOR
VITAL CAUSES OF OVERWEIGHT

1. Relax.
2. Set up a right and left finger signal for "yes" and "no."
3. Check with simple questions to which you know the answers. Do not consciously move index fingers. Let them move themselves. If movement is not discernible, repeat steps 1 and 2.
4. Ask questions requiring a "yes" and "no" answer to pinpoint year, place, person(s), and incident.

A PEEK INTO THE MEMORIES OF SOME
OVERWEIGHT PEOPLE

Many memories dredged up from the subconscious have a causative effect on overeating and are not pleasant memories.

They affect eating since they are unpleasant and beg to be compensated for with pleasure from some source such as food.

This woman, 39, did some dredging. What she found helped her to lose 76 pounds:

"All my life—from the time I was a little girl eight years old—my father said I was no good, the same as my real mother.

"I have felt inferior deep down inside, the bad one, the one who caused misery for everybody around me. When something would go wrong, it was my fault. When my brothers and sister were naughty, it was my fault. I was a bad example for them.

"Then throughout life when anything went wrong, I actually felt deep inside that it was my fault.

"How could anybody be so darn bad. I was terrible. It would be better if I wasn't around anymore.

"I retreated into fatness. If I was fat, I wouldn't have to go anyplace to cause trouble. . . ."

Sometimes it is the mother at whom memories point the overweight finger:

"I am struggling and I feel the struggle is nearly over. I am conscious and aware more often now of what this struggle really is. 'It' is my past life, the negative. It is not the natural me, with talents, smiles and capabilities that I possess.

"I am reacting instead of living. It is my mother's voice I am reacting to. She says, 'You are as rotten as your Dad.'

"So disappointed. This attitude is why I expect the negative. Mama must be exploded out of my spirit, so I can quit struggling and be what I am. Writing this as I feel helps to discharge some of the negative feelings."

This man, 45, suddenly remembered—without having to go through the finger raising procedure. Like a forgotten name, probe your memory, then relax, and it will pop into your mind when you least expect. Then write about it:

"It came to me one day that possibly my weight problem may have begun when I was a kid. My Dad was always nagging me at the dinner table. It was pure hell.

"I bolted my food as fast as I could so I could be excused. To this day I am still a fast eater. I was always a nervous wreck then. I had a bad eye blinking habit. I can well imagine this has something to do with the same problem."

Sometimes the experience that scars the personality does not involve a member of the family. Keep this in mind when you work your finger technique. "Was it a neighbor?" "Did it involve a schoolmate?" "Was it a storekeeper?"

> "The chubby little girl was looking in the window at the nice toys. The kindly, old proprietor (much like her own grandfather) invited her in to see the rest of the wonderful toys and 'something just for you—something very special.'
>
> "You'll say an event which occurred 50 years ago should not affect me now. Perhaps it wouldn't if it had been a cruel, brutal seduction by a criminal-type individual. This dear old gentleman was one of the town's leading merchants—pillar of the church and all that."

P.M. began to lose at the rate of ten pounds a month when she first began to record memories like these:

> "I'm twenty years old and I've been overweight or obese approximately twelve of those years. I was raised by children of the depression and was given more than an ample amount of food to eat. Hot meals three times a day, plenty to eat and overeat, and snacks whenever desired. My habits of eating were almost completely unrestrained by my mother, who is a complying person by nature. What I wanted I received within reason.
>
> "From earliest recollections I was never given physical love and only a small amount of emotional or mental love. My mother is passive, and her personality is overshadowed by the silent dominance of my father.
>
> "I must have felt a great deal of inner uncertainty about myself due to my family upbringing. So, I possibly could have turned to food as my only channel of security and warmth when very young."

Here's a young woman who had an easy time pinpointing the foods that caused her to gain and the period of her life when it happened. She weighed as much as 165 during her 26 years, quite an elevated weight for her scant five feet of height. But our program brought her down to 115. On the way down she wrote:

> "My problem of being overweight basically began when I was a teenager. I liked sweets and never thought of the consequences I would suffer. As a result of eating cake, candy, ice cream, etc., I developed a bad case of acne which required a lot of money and time to treat.
>
> "The more I was told I was 'fat,' the more I would eat. I didn't have any dates, but I had a lot of girlfriends. I hung around with a bad crowd because they accepted me as I was and never made fun of me."

Insight into one's inner emotional workings often provides some surprises.

One man reported he discovered he wasn't chewing his food; instead, he was swallowing it whole.

A wife found that she ate everytime her husband put her down—which was incessantly. She programed herself to respect herself more. Result: she didn't eat, she just left him.

"Overeating is related to an inner rage at having to grow up" was the way a man in his thirties described his insight. He realized he could never relax his guard against this.

Look for the breakthrough to come gradually—perhaps not as the word may lead you to believe. E.T., a 37-year old housewife reduced her weight from 158 to 130 in four months. Then she wrote:

"Now I walk with a better posture, holding my head erect. Men on the street turn around and look at me twice. People seem to be friendlier. I am more enthusiastic, have the desire to go and do things. I move faster and easier, do things with greater ease. No longer is shortness of breath noticeable. My back problem has not recurred since I began losing weight.

"I can't say I have confidence in myself and will be able to continue with these new ways and habits all my life—I have been disappointed too many times. But it's actually I, myself, who has been disappointing myself. No other person or thing is responsible. It seems that if it depends on me, I should be able to do it. Think, think, think—it's hard to change the bad habits of a life time."

People don't believe possible what hasn't happened. People don't believe it is possible to achieve perfect weight control—a MIRACLE.

Incidentally, E.T. went on to drop more unwanted pounds and became more and more confident of herself as the admiring glances multiplied.

THE IMPORTANCE OF CONFESSING TODAY FOR
YESTERDAY'S MISTAKES

The confessional, whether it takes place on a psychiatrist's couch or in a church, is always an enlightening procedure. The person who confesses usually feels a load has been lifted off his shoulders.

I hope that thinking, remembering, identifying and recording will become the overweight person's confessional. It not only takes a load off your shoulders but off your feet as well.

All over the Los Angeles area overweight people are confessing:

"I'm just beginning to know how frustrated I have been for years. How angry I am. How I haven't ever expressed it as anger, but only pain in my chest and hurt feelings.

"Two years ago I almost committed suicide. It would have been such an easy way out but one of the worst things a mother can do to her children. I resisted the temptation.

"Instead I asked my husband for a divorce, went on a diet, and went on the wagon.

"For six months I was in euphoria. I felt as though some one had literally let me out of jail. I was free. What a marvelous feeling. And I lost weight. Pounds. So easily.

"Sixty-two pounds later, I went to a studio party and fell off the wagon. An image of niceness that really wasn't true at all faded.

"My husband had a girlfriend three weeks after we were married. There were so many times I tried to get a divorce in those twenty-five years. Every two or three years we would have a crisis, and I would try to break free. He would insist on staying married, my mother would carry on, and he would change his ways for awhile. And I would feel less loved, less attractive, and more pain in the middle of my chest. And I would gain more weight until I was ashamed of myself and would find another doctor. This happened over and over again.

"At long last I have found I am mad, furious and sick of being used."

Confessing your inner thoughts is not easy. It takes a type of intestinal strength. But it gives you back just as much as it takes. You find you are better able to continue on the program of proper eating once you have released the emotional pressures within you.

Here are overweight people confessing:

"I resent my husband not setting a proper example for the kids."

"I see my parents only in passing. I feel guilty about not doing much work around the house."

"My grandparents could never quite understand why I preferred living with my mother and philandering father in the most abject poverty, when living with them would be living in abundance. They were always trying to fatten me up."

"My wife and I have had some good times together. We could laugh and talk and enjoy the same things together. But that person no longer exists. God, how I miss the person I once knew."

"I found myself pregnant and married the man. I never loved him. I eat because I don't have pleasures out of life, like a good sex life. . . ."

"I started to bottle up my sex drive. Then I started to bottle up other emotions. Soon I had built a strong brick wall of resentment, fear, and depression between myself and life."

"As a small child covers his eyes with his hands and plays hide and seek, so do I harbor more than one hundred pounds of excess weight, and cry out to all, 'Ha, ha, you can't see the real me.' If you can't see the real me, you cannot reject me. You cannot reject me because you don't know me. You can't see the real me, only the false front."

"Ah, Food, what a glorious, hideous substance you are . . . my joy, my downfall and my master. I hate you, yet I need you . . . I'm a nothing. No thing. No self-respect or strength. Help me, touch me, see me, love me. No, I won't let you. No one will penetrate my protective shell."

HOW TO REMOVE THE STING
FROM LETHAL THOUGHTS

Thoughts you allow to drive you to food are, in a way, destructive thoughts.

You may not always be capable of seeing their destructive nature. But certainly you know these thoughts are causing you to overeat, to be overweight, and therefore to live less than your normal life span.

Some of these thoughts are like slow suicide.

I am not a psychiatrist. You are not a psychiatrist. If you discover through writing that you have thoughts which now reveal themselves to be so despondent as to border on the suicidal, seek professional help. Of course, this would be a rarity.

Thinking about yourself, writing about yourself, confessing about the thoughts and ideas "bugging" you—these steps do not cause despondency. Rather, they permit the inner seething to surface, like pus in a boil.

There can be an emotional crisis, just as a body fever peaks, then the danger is over and healing takes place.

If you feel you are going through such a crisis, seek nearby professional help to see you through it.

When this woman wrote what you will now read, she was going through such a crisis. Writing helped to reveal it and possibly to stave off more rapid means of self-destruction than eating doughnuts:

> "To run away, oh what a wonderful thing to do—then I wouldn't have to face life or my children—then I wouldn't be here for them to torment, or have to take their calls. The only time they call is if they want something or are in trouble.
>
> "I'm so tired of giving, giving, giving. Why can't they realize I'm a human being too? Why must I give up my few pleasures just to help them out of a jam? I'm so tired.
>
> "I thought I had one good friend, then found she is just the same wants, wants, wants. I think they would take my blood if they could. I'm depressed, I'm tired, I'm nothing. Why can't I say 'no.'
>
> "I know my husband has to work these god-forsaken hours, but this loneliness is becoming too much for me. I can't read, or sew or crochet—my nerves are gone.
>
> "All I do is eat doughnuts—doughnuts and more doughnuts—so I grow fat. Who's here to care—I don't. This depression is growing worse—last week it wasn't too bad—I just continued eating. This week it's worse—I'm eating and eating, and I look it . . .
>
> "I need help. I need help. . ."

Don't be frightened at the thoughts you dredge up by thinking and writing. Hidden, they are sapping your life energy. You eat to compensate for the loss of this life energy. Exposed, these thoughts are no longer able to do their dirty work. Think about it. Then. . . .

Write and the pressure to overeat will begin to diminish.

Write and the "quiet desperation" will tend to dissolve.

Write and the barrier to a fuller life, be that barrier pounds or pangs, will begin to disappear.

HOW SPENDING TIME WITH YOURSELF BRINGS YOU GREATER EMOTIONAL HEALTH AND FREEDOM FROM OBSESSION WITH FOOD

"I'm going to have something to eat."

That's all it takes. That thought. And away you go.

It is not *you* originating that thought. It's your subconscious mind. It is an automatic thought. Programing.

Now you know the difference. Now when you think that thought, instead of trying to fight it, and losing the battle, you study it, understand it and win the battle.

I hope you will think about yourself and write.

Allow yourself time to meditate each day in a peaceful, quiet setting. Think about your overweight problem. How did it begin? Why did it begin? Why has it continued for so many years, perhaps all your life? Why have you repeatedly failed or let yourself down? What special situations or rationalizations contribute to or prolong your overweight problem? What experiences both past and recent relate to your problem? What are the most significant and difficult aspects of your physical and emotional being? Then write about it.

D.H. had been a widow for four years. "I had no interest in anything except my own sorrow." She never connected the sorrow to what was happening on the scale. Finally, when her weight and blood pressure rose to dangerous levels, she came into the program.

In 14 weeks she not only weighed 30 pounds less, but her blood pressure was 130 over 90, not bad for a 56-year old person. Her sorrow gave way to sociability. Today, she's dressing fashionably and going places.

An inner strength is developed in this program. Perhaps, I should say that it has always been there but somehow the program dusts it off, oils it up, and permits it to go to work.

C.B. was recently divorced. That's not easy for a woman to take at 48, and it shook her up emotionally. She began to lean on food for her emotional security. She soon weighed 188, which at 5'2", made her a well-rounded person indeed. She became very loud and agitated, perhaps as a cover-up to her insecurity and depression. Five months into the program she weighed 135. She was more subdued, warm, and friendly. Her son had moved away, another shock for her, but she took it in stride. Last I saw C.B. she was dressed attractively and busy socially. Her inner strength was making her a well rounded person in the proper sense.

It's not the weight loss that produces changes as much as it is the insight. Take C.L., 25, engaged to a man several years her junior. She had a serious, bed confining accident. She brooded about it—and overate about it. Her relationship with her fiance was faltering. I saw her when her weight was 170 and rising. She appeared to be 40. She programed herself well, thought about her attitudes and emotions, wrote, read what she wrote and thought some more.

Soon she realized she was in control of herself. She could take things her fiancé said without over-reacting. She could go to the restaurant and enjoy eating simple meat and salad dishes. In six weeks some 30 pounds had disappeared. But what appeared was yet more impressive: self-assuredness, calmness, efficiency, a happy temperament. She and her fiancé are now married.

Here are some tips to make this very important part of the weight control program more meaningful and productive of eating habit changes for you:

- Words, phrases or sentences you may consider trivial can be the most significant. Capture them all on paper.
- Do not concern yourself with grammar or sentence structure. No one other than you need read what you write.
- Do it now. Procrastination will permit the valuable insight to drift out of sight.
- Express your feelings and emotions freely. Don't edit what the subconconscious mind sends up to you.
- Ask yourself feeling-triggering questions. "How do I really feel about so and so?" "What is my real attitude toward that problem?" And so forth.
- Read your material over and over again. Reading aloud helps. Let what you have written trigger other thoughts. There is no such thing as a final thought.
- Question yourself thoroughly about everything you have written. Ask yourself "How?" "Why?" "What?" "When?" "Where?" Be firm with yourself. Don't allow any questions to go unanswered. The subconscious can throw all sorts of diversions at you to protect its secrets. See through it. Let it all "hang out"—easily.
- Don't struggle—eventually to give up or backslide. Don't battle or fight yourself—losing more than you attain. Don't reproach or downgrade yourself. Instead, learn to be your own listening post, your own sounding board. Learn to be a weight thinker, a weight loser, a weight doer.
- Hours after you write, thoughts may pop into your mind about your overweight problem and the causes behind it. Don't assure yourself you can remember. Jot it down instantly. Just a few notes at a given moment will help trigger your memory later; then you can expand these notes.
- Program yourself to write about yourself. Know it will "untangle the wires" and eventually lead to self-awareness, self-understanding and self-discovery.

The Meat of Chapter 10

"I cause myself to become discouraged when the scales don't move." The scales will move when you move mentally. Read what others are discovering about themselves. It triggers you to discover more about yourself.

Learn how to probe your subconscious for hidden causes and excuses using the finger signal method. Move mentally. Move toward self-discovery. Write about whatever you discover. If what you write about sounds like True Confessions, remember that confessing, telling all, takes a load off you. What better time to sit down and think some serious thoughts than right now. Write now!

11

TEN STEPS TO A GREAT NEW SLENDER LIFE

Appetizer for Chapter 11

I apologize. I have been long winded about a slenderizing program that is actually very simple. In this chapter I sum it up for you. It boils down into ten easy steps. Not dance steps, but just as much fun.

If all the deaths due to cancer were eliminated, the average life span of the people in this country would be extended two years.

If all the deaths due to overweight and obesity were eliminated, the average life span of the people in this country would be extended seven years.

Yes, being overweight in the United States takes more than triple the toll of cancer. This means that more than 60 million overweight Americans should become aware to resolve the problem now.

There is no escape. The clock is ticking away. Pretend you're blasted off to Skylab where everyone experiences weightlessness. You are still an overweight person facing the same health problems.

The place is here. The time is now. You have the best opportunity while this book is in your hands to solve your problem and enjoy your rightful share of healthy, happy years.

Until now you have been given a way that we'll soon look back upon as belonging to the Dark Ages: Diet.

What a tragedy that you have had to subject yourself to this torture to no permanent avail!

You're within ten steps of freedom and never having to go on a diet again. They are so very easy, especially compared to dieting, that you will wonder why the word is still in the dictionary.

I will list these ten steps now. Then I will devote a sub-heading to each one (except the last which will be covered in the next and final chapter) so you can have the steps summarized in capsule form.

1. Switch to high protein, low carbohydrate, low fat foods.

2. Consult with your physician about your plans, soliciting his counsel and assistance.

3. Set a goal for your new profile in weight and/or measurements.

4. Turn on your awareness about food, your attitude toward it, your enjoyment of it.

5. Identify the circumstances or emotional causes which trigger false appetites within you.

6. Write about yourself, your problems, and your solutions.

7. Develop the skill of attaining a deep state of relaxation of body and mind.

8. Program yourself, while relaxed, for improving your self-image, eating properly, responding more positively, and reaching your goal.

9. Engage in more physical activity and exercise.

10. Shift to the maintenance program when you achieve your goal.

STEP 1: THE FOOD PROGRAM: HIGH PROTEIN, LOW CARBOHYDRATE, LOW FAT

An internationally known nutritionist at Georgetown University has identified a disease he calls "affluent malnutrition." As societies become more affluent, they change their eating habits two basic ways: (1) They eat too much. (2) They eat more expensive, processed foods, losing out on vital trace nutrients and a proper balance of minerals and vitamins. True. And I add, "They also eat more sugar."

Do you know there is sugar in such packaged foods as a noodles and cheese dinner, a lasagne dinner, chili con carne?

American food processors commonly determine how much sugar to include in a product by having a group of ordinary consumers as their official tasters. These men, women and children say which samples taste best.

No test is made of which samples are best for you, only which samples taste best to taste buds that are being programed yearly for more and more sweetness.

Can you see the direction processed foods are taking? Is there any wonder that the obesity statistics are so frighteningly high?

Cows that graze in verdant pastures are attracted to those grasses which are most nutritious. Can you imagine where they would be if the entire pasture was sprinkled with sugar?

I indict sugar as the overweight people's Public Enemy No. 1.

Next is bread, and its family of family fatteners. Bread was once called the staff of life. Today, the stuff of life is out of the staff of life. What is included after taking out the germ of the wheat is a farce. The truth is that "enriched" bread is still "depleted" bread compared to the fresh, stone ground, whole wheat flour our forebears used.

So we smear butter and jam and other goo on this worthless, tasteless white stuff and thus compound the felony.

For the Hall of Food Infamy, I nominate flour and all of its cake, cracker, cookie and cereal cousins as the overweight people's Public Enemy No. 2.

If we overweights would lock up these two culprits for life, we would all live longer.

Well, enough said about them. Let's concentrate on what is nourishing instead of what's fattening.

You know you can enjoy normal satisfying portions of beef, veal, lamb, chicken, squab and turkey.

The world of fish and seafood is yours to enjoy and better food for your body is hard to find. Buy it fresh, frozen or canned.

You know you can enjoy eggs, lower fat content cheeses, and low fat dairy products.

You know the best low carbohydrate fruits and vegetables to select.

Drink at least eight full glasses of liquid per day.

Review Chapter 3 for the "yes" and "no" foods.

As the ads say, "Get to know what good is."

The divorce rate in the U.S. is very high. I have seen some marriages fail when one of the partners gained self-confidence and lost weight. But I have seen far more marriages saved by one or both of the partners slimming down.

D.D. came to the office looking morose and dejected. Her despondent state was far more noticeable than her weight, 138. Her husband who, she said, was very figure conscious, was making remarks about "letting herself go" and he was becoming less interested in her.

"He says he doesn't enjoy placing his arm around me and grabbing a handful of flesh."

Some four months later, weighing 108 pounds, D.D. was sparkling, talkative, vivacious and outgoing. Her marriage was as strong as it used to be and she was a wit wiser. "He likes women lean and slender and if his wife isn't attractive to him, someone else will be."

STEP 2: MEDICAL AIDS YOUR PHYSICIAN MAY SUPPLY

Here are some of the medical checks I do for my patients. Naturally, I weigh them, check their blood pressure and pulse. Since I have previously taken their medical history, there are other questions I may ask and tests I may want to make relative to past problems as they progress.

I prescribe therapeutic vitamins and mineral supplements at breakfast with emphasis on B-complex vitamins which I consider important to weight and fat loss. I recommend to my patients a minimum of 250 milligrams of Vitamin C four times a day and at least 200 International Units of Vitamin E at supper time.

I also prescribe a hunger suppressant to assist my patients while they are reprograming for normal hunger control.

I have been amazed at the lack of information on the part of those who criticize the benefits of hunger suppressants in hunger control. I have observed thousands of patients who have used them. When the patient is properly instructed as to the reasons and need for this medication as an adjunct to control hunger for a limited period of time, the results are excellent.

Some patients need a thyroid supplement as supportive medication, others a diuretic, still others a temporary laxative (I favor milk of magnesia).

These are matters for your own physician to decide.

Step 1 is to eliminate all those "foods" that are adding to your weight problems—the fats, sweets and starches. Substitute nutritious proteins. If you haven't already done so, do it now. Eat to be well, not to swell.

Step 2 is to visit your physician and explain your plans. Solicit his support and watchful eye. Consult with him about your weight problem and seek his advice to help you with Step 3.

STEP 3: SET A GOAL FOR PROFILE CONTROL

"Doctor, I can't wait to reach my goal."

"You must develop patience."

If Benjamin Franklin was right when he said, "He that can have patience can have what he will," then impatience must be the spawner of failures.

Men and women who can't wait to reach their weight goal, usually don't.

Patience is power.

To set a weight goal or measurement goal is important. To give it an unreasonable time limit is to exhibit impatience.

If you had a choice of the following two sets of circumstances, which would you choose?—

1. To reach your weight goal in four months and remain at that perfect weight for the rest of your life.
2. To reach your weight goal in two months and gain back all the fat you lost in another two months.

Allow yourself time to acquire the measurements and looks for which you aim. You are going to be slender and attractive for a long, long time.

Sometimes it doesn't take many excess pounds to ruin a life.

M.J., 26, was a teacher in a private school. Although she weighed only 122, not many pounds in excess for her 5'1" height, it made her insecure socially.

To compensate, she acted very snooty and conceited. This doesn't enhance one's professional relations, also she was unpopular with her colleagues despite her talents in music, drama and poetry.

She was a very attractive girl, but confessed she had never dated very much. In two weeks she gave up nine pounds. It required four months to drop another eight pounds and reach her 105 pound goal.

Meanwhile, she began dating. "It's about time," she commented good humoredly. Good humor was her trademark now instead of conceit. She invited her fellow teachers and friends to her house for parties. I was very impressed with the differences a few pounds could make.

Another great change after only a few pounds was experienced by M.L., a 32-year-old divorcee with three children. She wasn't happy having to return to work because of her scant divorce settlement. She was per-

petually tired, depressed and looked much older than her years. At 5'4",
the 123 pounds did not seem to be her problem. Yet, when she shed ten
pounds (it required five months), she perked up as though a load had been
removed. She began dating a great fellow who was good to her children
and then, due to the remarkable changes in her, he started on the program
to shed a few pounds, too.

Miracles can't be measured in time, pounds or inches alone. One
of the most important characteristics of the subconscious mind is
"feelings." It is emotional with each and every one.

Here are some typical weights, goals, and times of attainment:

Sex	Weight First Visit	Goal	Weight Final Visit	Pounds Lost	Months Elapsed
Male	201	130	143	58	14
Male	178	140	139	39	20
Female	220	125	155	65	28
Male	276	160	168	108	21
Female	141	120	123	18	4
Female	157	125	126	31	3
Male	233	150	165	68	5
Female	139	115	118	21	1
Female	180	125	125	55	5
Female	170	120	115	55	13

Note that several had not reached their goal when I last saw
them. This does not mean that they failed. I'll give odds that most
leveled themselves out at their target weight or close to it.

When you set a weight or measurement goal and program
yourself (Chapter 8) to reach it, it's more difficult to prevent
yourself from reaching it than it actually is to reach it. Example:
You are programed to breathe. It's impossible to stop breathing.

Note, too, although it required one patient 13 months to lose
55 pounds, another reached an equivalent goal within 5 months.
Can you say the person who required the longer time failed? Of
course not. They both set a goal and reached it.

If you keep a weight or measurement chart showing your
progress, progress toward your goal is the key. Progress measured
in time is interesting, but progress versus no progress is much more
than just interesting. *It is vital.*

STEP 4: TURN ON YOUR AWARENESS
OF HOW FOOD TURNS YOU ON

A woman in her forties came to see me. She was separated from her husband, a psychologist. She weighed 140 on my scale and measured 5'2". She said her overweight problem was the reason for her marital problem.

"My husband says he's not proud of me. He can't look up to me. I'm too fat. We've been apart five months, and he complains that I have not done anything to win him back."

I was puzzled. "Can he turn love on and off if you're ten or fifteen pounds one way or the other?"

"I think that's just an excuse. He has problems. I've always given in to him except for the weight. Still, I don't seem to be able to do anything right. No matter how I have tried, I don't suit him."

"Do you suit yourself?"

"I don't have confidence in myself. I want my husband back, but I don't think I will feel the same about him. Still, I don't feel I can go out and meet others on a woman-to-man basis."

"Where can you go for more self-confidence?" I asked. "The grocery store, the city dump, a garage sale?"

"I will probably acquire confidence when my weight goes down. My husband says I'm terribly, terribly obese. My confidence is there but my weight is blocking it."

"Is your weight blocking your confidence? Or are *you* blocking it?"

"Do you think I'm doing the same thing as my husband? Using my weight as an excuse?"

I share this brief conversation with you to illustrate how quickly it is possible to gain insight into yourself once you begin to think about yourself.

Make a two pronged probe into your life. One prong throws light on exactly what triggers your false appetite. Those are the Pavlov bells we talked about. Note where, what, when, how and why you eat. Implement the 25 tips for fooling those bells listed in Chapter 2.

The second prong throws light on your innermost feelings and attitudes.

What is the connection between your mood and your food?

STEP 5: ADJUST YOUR MOOD
AND YOU ADJUST YOUR FOOD

A young woman, 22, describes her craving for certain foods:

"I never keep cookies around, although I often dream about them at night. Sometimes I dream about chocolate cake, sometimes feasts. But I never have enough cookies to satisfy me.

"Once I awoke in the middle of the night with an intense craving for cookies. Creeping downstairs to the kitchen, I examined the contents of the cupboards. Rows of spices labeled 'Miriam Ross.' (She shares the house with me and understands my night wanderings well.) A box of corn flakes labeled 'Miriam Ross.' A bag of marshmallows labeled 'Miriam Ross.' And various other 'goodies' bearing the same label.

"Marshmallows are nice in the middle of the night. Or any time when Miriam is not around. She becomes quite angry if she counts them and finds five missing. I offer to buy her some more. She agrees. A ten-ounce bag costs 29¢. She labels them when I give them to her. I particularly enjoy them when they say 'Miriam Ross.' Otherwise, I don't really care much for marshmallows. I relive this occasionally."

Reliving this occasionally led her to reflecting upon teenage days. Her mother was a model, was very busy and had little time to cook. What does a growing 13 or 14 year old do under these conditions? She visits friends and "grubs" snacks. Now she recalls all the conniving she did to "grub" other people's food.

Being aware of her nightly forays now led to understanding them. Understanding them led to controlling them easily through reprograming.

The path to obesity is lined with boredom, frustration, anxiety, insecurity, guilt, and unfulfilled needs.

Sometimes you cannot control the cause of the worry, but you can always control its connection to your salivary glands. P.J. was married to a racing car driver. As he drove, she was driven to gorging herself, to divert her mind from his danger.

One pound shy of 200, she came to the office and started on the program. Perhaps she didn't develop a philosophy about life and death, but she disconnected eating from worrying. In six months, she crocheted a wardrobe, and lost 53 pounds.

There is a favorite maxim among physicians: Listen to the patient long enough and the patient will reveal whatever is wrong. Thus many doctors make time to listen to their patients. I listen. But if the patient listens to himself, too, that's much better; especially when the cause is a problem that activates the appetite.

"If you straighten out your emotional problems you will straighten out your weight problem." So spoke P.R.'s psychiatrist. Her child had been killed in an auto accident and she went into a state of psychological paralysis for about a year.

I feel it could have gone on much longer if she had not begun to think about what she was doing to herself. She came into the weight control program at 160. You should have seen her then. She sat in the reception room like a mummy with a long face—jeans, t-shirt, bare feet. She never spoke to anyone, including me.

When she began to speak, it was only after several false starts on the program, with periods of a month or more when we thought we saw the last of her. Then she began talking about the accident and how numb she was to life and to her husband's touch.

With the flow of words (which I couldn't convince her to set down on paper but why push my luck), came a change in her whole personality and appearance. She not only kept her appointments, but came in between to check her weight, always cordial, warm, friendly and talkative. Her outlook changed miraculously as verbalization uprooted false "appetite triggers." She last weighed in at 142 and although her desired weight was 130, I had no doubt P.R. would make it.

Think.
Identify.
Understand.
Write. . . .

STEP 6: WHEN YOU BECOME A WRITER, YOU BECOME A RIGHT-ER

As you know by now, if I had to put priorities on the ten major steps in this program, I would place *writing* very close to the top.

When you write, food intake wrongs are righted.

If you don't have a small pad and pencil or pen near you right now, how can you write now?

Please be ready to write at all times. Keep a small memo pad in your purse or pocket. Keep it on your night table or under your pillow when you retire.

Be prepared for a sudden thought that could change everything for the better.

"Today, I thought no one answered my resumés because I was old and fat. The resumés show my age as 47 and my weight as 125. I actually weigh 137. At 5'5" I'm not grossly overweight on the resumé. This couldn't be the reason. I guess when anything makes me unhappy or doesn't go well, I blame my weight."

No big thing. But this little piece of insight, recorded on a little pad with a little stub of a pencil, led to further insights and to this woman's loss of twenty pounds in the next three months.

Insight pays off handsomely not only in a pound of flesh today, but in a permanent resistance to those excess pounds of flesh in the future.

There are cases of obesity due to physical inactivity, to metabolic or glandular imbalances, and to genetic or hereditary causes. For each of these, there are a hundred cases due to overprotective parents, philandering spouses, dismal self-images, and similar emotional origins.

"I've never talked or written about myself before," L.J. confessed to me. Her husband was a manager of an auto repair shop, while she worked as a secretary in a law firm. "It's extremely difficult to 'bare' myself. The more I hurt, the more I keep it inside."

The more she kept it inside, the more food she shoved inside her. Now at 5'1" she weighed 149 pounds.

Then she began thinking about those "hurts" she was burying with food, and began to write and talk about herself. Her weight dropped 20 pounds in six weeks and she soon reached her goal of 115. "After I set it down on paper," she said later, "it felt so good."

The good news is, obesity due to emotional causes is curable.

The cure starts with thinking and identifying, then proceeds through writing, and finally to. . . .

STEP 7: RELAXATION—THE DOORWAY
TO YOUR PROGRAMABLE MIND

So often you hear, "When I stopped smoking, I gained weight." Well, it doesn't have to work that way. In this program, if you stop smoking, you don't gain as you program yourself to eat properly. If you feel you must chew instead of puff, think about yourself and don't overeat.

> Take P.W. When he stopped smoking, he joined the beef trust—added more than thirty pounds. When he first consulted me about his problem he had both—the smoking habit had returned (1½ packs a day) and the weight habit also. Well, P.W. learned self-hypnotism—the art of relaxing and programing the mind. He used his mental screen a few times a day, seeing himself a slim, non-smoker. It required two months to drop the smoking, and another month to drop the poundage, but he completed the program free of both.

You know best which of the techniques described in Chapter 8 relax you more rapidly and deeply. Develop skill at relaxation. It is Step 7.

If you have a cassette, you can make your own relaxation tape—talking to yourself in a soothing voice, inducing a deep state of comfort and tranquility of body and mind.

In this state your subconscious mind is at your service. It is ready to be reprogramed.

Step 8 is. . . .

REPROGRAMING YOUR MIND FOR MENTAL
AND ALIMENTAL CONTROL

"I am fully satisfied with smaller portions. I enjoy protein foods and no longer need sweets, starches and fats. I eat more slowly and derive more satisfaction from every mouthful."

These are the sounds of programing.

"I see myself slender and popular. I see myself being successful at whatever I do. I see myself confident, self-assured, capable."

These are the sights and pictures of programing.

They are creating exactly what they say or see—with no ands, ifs, or buts.

There are many uses for programing. If you are not motivated to program yourself, you can program yourself to be so motivated. How? Well, you asked the question so you must be curious enough to attempt it once or twice. Use those few relaxed times to see yourself sitting in a chair, relaxing, programing and accomplishing anything you desire.

It will soon be your favorite chair.

You can program yourself to eat at certain times and to eat properly.

You can program yourself to enjoy non-fattening foods and to be unmoved by fattening foods.

You can program yourself to see the good side of life instead of the morbid side.

You can program yourself right out of fears, anxieties, and other negative emotions and smack into exhilerating, uplifting and enthusiastic moods.

You can program yourself to reach goals—including the goal of physical attractiveness.

You can program yourself to derive more fun out of everything you do.

The skills developed in this program stand you in good stead forever. F.A. transformed herself from 139 to 117 during her few months on the program, from unemployed to employed with a promotion the second week, and from a quiet, dull personality to an interesting, vivacious person.

But a big dividend occurred years later. She married, became pregnant, and after delivery weighed a pound less than she did nine months before.

STEP 9: WEIGHT AND FAT LOSS
IS ACCELERATED BY PHYSICAL ACTIVITY

Step 9 of the program is the stepping up of physical activity.

The best exercise of all is lifting yourself up by your bootstraps. Begin thinking about yourself and you do it naturally. Begin writing about yourself and you may be unable to stop. Begin exercising, even though it's like pulling teeth. Eventually the going becomes easier and easier.

K.D., 43 and a housewife, felt she had plenty of activity making beds, cooking, and cleaning. But she forced herself to do a few minutes of prescribed exercises. Then she experienced a physical breakthrough. She began to enjoy doing them. Exercised while waiting for me in the office. She learned yoga and taught it to my nurses. K.D. had set a goal of 125 when she began the program at 165. She reached her goal in seven months.

The more active you are, the more energy you burn. The more energy you burn, the less your body stores. 3,500 calories of stored energy weighs one pound.

Learn to golf. Begin playing tennis again. Bowl more frequently. Buy a Ping-Pong table for the basement or spare room or string up a badminton or volleyball net in the backyard.

Walk more. Dance more. Swim more. Jog more.

Instead of pushing the elevator button, push yourself to walk up a few flights, or down.

Some exercises set you up for the day like sit-ups and push-ups. So-called isometric exercises improve muscle tone. To do them you push with one arm and resist with the other. You can also improve muscle tone with finger, arm, leg, muscle and back movements.

Invent your own exercises. Never strain or fatigue yourself but go a little further each day, challenging your body gently.

Start gradually. If you pour yourself into calisthenics too enthusiastically, muscles that previously have not been used consistently will rebel and give you a "stiff" time. Proceed at your own pace. Stop, rest, continue.

As you become accustomed to exercising, you can increase the rate at which you do them. This provides greater stimulation to the circulatory and respiratory systems. Check your breathing and heart rate. These should be normal ten minutes after you stop exercising.

As you continue your exercises, you will feel their tonic effect. Daily work will be easier. You will have more energy reserve at the end of the day. Also, your posture will improve. Your skin will become more radiant. There will be more spring in your step. You will appear and feel years younger.

You are a protein eater. You are a weight thinker, a weight loser.

You have straightened out your eating habits and your emotional posture through reprograming. You are an active person. You are shedding weight and fat. And then . . .

You reach your goal.

You are slender, physically attractive, healthier.

Now what?

Do you go back on that yo-yo of lose and regain?

Not on your life. You take Step 10. You insure you will never again have the overweight nightmare.

You embark on the maintenance program for permanent fun out of life.

Meat of Chapter 11

This chapter has been essentially a review of the program so you can grasp its really simple procedures. Although I have broken it down into ten steps, I can probably give you the meat of the program in three words: 1. Protein 2. Self-analysis 3. Reprograming. However, even though your weight goal is reached, the program does not end here. Save Chapter 12 until that great day arrives. Or peek now at the maintenance program, if you must. It is Step 10.

12

HOW TO MAINTAIN YOUR BODY
AT ITS ATTRACTIVE BEST
WITHOUT A SECOND THOUGHT

The Appetizer for Chapter 12

The first eleven chapters covered the time required to reach your perfect weight. This chapter covers the rest of your lengthened life. It tells you how to maintain your ideal weight. You will be expanding your menus without expanding your girth. You may eat some bread and ice cream. But you never stop thinking about you know who.

This chapter should be read after you have shed all the fat and weight you desire.

Let me tell you at the outset you will be able to restore a number of foods on your maintenance program. These are carbohydrates and fats that were either prohibited or restricted on your weight and fat loss program. We will discuss the details of this in a page or two.

Remember, however, these carbohydrates and fats are the valves for weight control. Eat more of them, you gain. Eat less of them, you stop gaining. Eat even less, you drop pounds.

This control of carbohydrates and fats is very easy for you now. The reasons are:

- You are now keenly aware of your eating habits. Sweets and starches, fats and oils can no longer pull the wool over your eyes.

- You are now keenly aware of your own feelings and emotions, how they tend to express and compensate through food, and how they can once again program false hunger if you let them.
- You are programed to enjoy proteins. Fats and carbohydrates no longer have the hold on you they once had.

You have reached your desired weight. You can now turn the carbohydrate and fat valve back on—slowly. Here is how.

HOW TO ADD FATS AND CARBOHYDRATES
WITHOUT ADDING POUNDS

Add the carbohydrate foods first that are best for your body. I guess you know I am talking about vegetables. Remember, you previously cut your intake of vegetables until your weight loss was assured. Now you can:

- Add different vegetables.
- Increase portions slowly, cautiously.

Here are some varieties of preferred vegetables you can add to vegetable choices:

Tomatoes	Brussels Sprouts
Peas	Egg Plant
Snow Peas	Zucchini
Turnips	Soy Beans

Drag your feet on lima beans, corn, lentils, navy beans, kidney beans and other starchy vegetables. These are definitely *not* part of your maintenance program.

I know many are holding your breath, hoping I'll give you the green light on potatoes. No way. If lima beans appear on your plate occasionally when you eat out, you are unlikely to reprogram yourself to accept lima beans. However, if you re-admit potatoes, potatoes will likely appear on your plate every day. Potatoes can be a way of life if you let them—an overweight life.

If you can place potatoes in the same category as cauliflower or asparagus—that is, an occasional choice—then I say go ahead and have a baked or boiled potato once a week.

You can also have a thin pat of margarine (poly-unsaturated) with it.

Make potatoes a habit if you wish (never home fried, hashed brown, or french fried) but make them a Sunday habit or a Friday or Saturday night habit.

Here are other additions you can make as you embark on your maintenance program:

- Other oils (besides safflower) with vinegar as dressing for salads, lightly applied.
- Two slices of bread per day.
- Up to three jiggers of alcoholic beverage, providing you deduct one slice of bread or one piece of fruit for each jigger.

Other oils can now be added lightly and cautiously to salad dressing. If the scale doesn't shudder from the impact, you can be less parsimonious. Understand this: you must always keep a wary eye pealed for oils and fats, sweets and starches.

The two slices of bread per day now permitted on the maintenance program will nearly double your carbohydrate intake compared to the weight and fat loss program.

So will two jiggers of alcoholic beverage.

That's why I couple them. Take your pick. Add both the bread and the liquor and you mandate a weight gain. Some days you may prefer the bread, toasted with thinly spread margarine for breakfast. Other days, you might feel sociable and want to hoist a couple.

The choice is yours. But never must the twain meet in the same 24-hour period.

I'LL TRADE YOU A PIECE OF FRUIT
FOR A SLICE OF BREAD

You take the fruit.

I'll take the bread.

I can handle it. My weight is well under the height-weight tables.

I say the limit is still one piece of fruit a day or one five-ounce glass of juice. Fruit has more nourishment than bread, especially fresh or frozen fruit. It has minerals, vitamins and enzyme material. You may wish to slice it into halves or thirds to spread the enjoyment all day.

Have another orange or apple or peach or pear and skip one slice of bread. Or have a third piece of fruit and cancel out the second slice of bread.

Of course, if you must have two slices of bread, you're limited to one piece of fruit. And, perchance you find yourself eating three slices of bread, don't shake my tree.

HOW TO: BALANCE CARBOHYDRATE INTAKE THROUGH FRUIT AND BREAD

The limit of total pieces of fruit and bread is three—

Fruit	Bread	Total Daily Intake
0	3	3
1	2	3
2	1	3
3	0	3

MAINTENANCE STILL MEANS HIGH PROTEIN, LOW FAT, LOW CARBOHYDRATE FOODS

Remember, you have not been on a diet. You have lost weight and fat on a program. You certainly are not going on a diet now.

You are going to have even more gustatory enjoyment on this maintenance program—fun with roasts, chops, steaks, filets, racks, ribs, and rumps; fun with fish and fowl; fun with egg dishes and cheeses galore.

You can be more lenient in your choice of meats, still cutting off excess fat, perhaps enjoying organ meats more frequently or loin of pork occasionally, where previously you had to be extra cautious.

You still cast a wary eye about for fat and sugar, but just as we added the two slices of bread and a few more vegetables, you can add some item occasionally that you enjoy.

One example would be ice cream. It is a national favorite. So have a large scoop or two small scoops once a week. Do it the way you added the potato to your menu—once a week, not as a regularly available food. (Or else!)

Some items can be added on a daily basis. Gelatin dessert, for instance, or a slice of bacon (crisp, dry), or non-fat milk in your coffee.

Add. Then weigh. You may be able to add again.

Or, you may have to subtract.

YOUR WEIGHT WILL RETURN READILY IF YOU INVITE IT

Backsliding is a common occurrence. It usually happens when there's a crisis or a change. You change your living pattern and your weight changes, too. What happens is that the change or crisis erases correct programing, if you permit, then you must reinforce that correct programing. You'll notice yourself saying, "Today is different. It is OK if I gorge myself today. Tomorrow I'll return to normal patterns." Of course, tomorrow drags its feet.

"Tomorrow is another day . . . I'll eat wisely then." That's what M.C. told herself on a tour that included 37 states. "But I just had to enjoy southern barbeques. After all I may never return. In Virginia it was candied yams. In Maine, lobster with lots of butter. In Vermont, pancakes and maple syrup. And how do you refuse relatives who want to show how well they eat—every meal a seven course banquet?"

M.C. acquired 13 unwanted pounds on that trip and I acquired a repeat patient.

"Here I am again, Doctor," said Jean as she walked in. "I guess I'm not the first to return. I just couldn't handle the situation at college. The social competition. Pressure in courses. I became upset. The people I called my friends just took advantage of me. I had no one to turn to. So I turned to food."

"Don't you call yourself a friend? Can't you trust yourself? Won't you help yourself?" I never expected to see this young woman again. Jean was a splendid patient on the program less than a year ago and shed weight from 165 to 128 in just three summer months. Now her weight was up to 156.

"I've taken a job selling clothes. I like it. I meet people. I discovered many things about myself in the past year. I realize I must stand on my own two feet. I'm not a baby. My parents spoil me. I don't want that anymore. I want to be independent and make my own decisions."

"Do you want to be a big person?"

"I can't see myself the way I am. I want to be smaller physically yet build up my self-confidence. I know the more independent I become, the greater my self-confidence will become."

"I admire you for your ability and capability. You have the potential for being one of the most beautiful and important people, unless you prefer to concern yourself with minor embarrassments and other people's failings." She shook her head. "Whatever goal you set, you will reach."

Jean came back into the program again with her goal, 125 pounds. In eight weeks she reached it.

No, she wasn't the only returnee. Hardly a week passes without seeing a familiar face, slightly puffed since the last time I saw it. However, scores continually graduate to the maintenance program and I never see them again.

I often wonder what happened to some of the unfinished stories.

What happened to the beautiful 25-year old girl who was a cold fish to her husband. He wanted children. But she wanted no part of him. Then she dropped 30 pounds on the program and they began going to dances every Saturday night.

What happened to the department store executive, a charming woman, who won awards as top saleswoman? Then she decided she was working her life away, lost 20 pounds and quit her job.

What happened to the 187 pound nervous young woman who at the age of 26 never had an orgasm? She threatened suicide, so her husband sent her to a psychiatrist. The psychiatrist referred her to me. She dropped about 50 pounds and they adopted a baby.

What happened to the supermarket check-out girl who had such terrible facial acne, her young husband divorced her? She dropped 25 pounds and her complexion became like peaches and cream.

What happened to the wife of a commercial pilot who ate to while away the time whenever he was away? Then she programed herself out of about 40 pounds, learned to fly, and bought her own plane.

I receive feedback via other patients about many of the interesting people who come to my office. But so many stories go unfinished.

Medical research has shown that overweight persons have: (1)

abnormally high levels of circulating insulin, and (2) abnormally low levels of circulating growth hormone.

When such an overweight person loses weight, insulin falls closer to a normal level.

BUT, the loss of weight does not affect the growth hormone for six to eight months. That is why so many people regain lost weight so easily.

The person who becomes slim must stand constant guard over their new found profile for at least a year.

Then as the circulating growth hormone gradually moves up toward a more normal level, the maintenance program can become more relaxed.

The patients who come back to see me usually have run into some difficult problems in life. Similar to Jean, with her new college experience, they return to the comforts of an old friend, "Fatty" Carbohydrate, only to find that it only compounds the problem.

I have found that these patients usually benefit by their first success. They know what the program is all about. They go off fats and carbohydrates and on to proteins. They think and write and reprogram themselves. Quicker'n you can say "poly-unsaturated," they reach their slender goal again.

Now, there is no need to slip back and have to go through the weight and fat loss program again. The answer is to think and write the very day you detect yourself compensating for some emotion or feeling by eating a chocolate sundae, or a pizza or another unhealthy fat, sweet or starch.

The moment you turn the hot, white light of your own scrutiny on such goings on, detect and understand your emotional requirements, reprogram to fill the personality void or imbalance, the urge to fill your mouth and belly with fat-making junk will turn tail and disappear.

HOW TO: STOP EATING BINGES IN THEIR TRACK!

1. Recognize you are on an eating binge.
2. Ask yourself why? How do you feel? Why are you running to food? What else can you do instead?
3. Write about these thoughts immediately. Study them later again. Program new thoughts. Jot these down, also.
4. Do several relaxation and reprograming sessions. See yourself remaining

on the maintenance program. See yourself doing what must and can be done to solve your basic emotional problems, and to restore your positivity and success-oriented self-image.

25 RECIPES FOR "ENJOYING" AND "MAINTAINING"

Here are additional recipes to illustrate the great dining you can experience without budging the scale one ounce upward.

The 25 recipes I shared with you in Chapter 3 are, of course, still appropriate for your maintenance program. But now you can add a gourmet flair here and there.

For instance, on the pages ahead, you will see "garnish with olives," "add bitter chocolate to gravy," "serve on toasted whole wheat bread," "sprinkle bacon on top." These would be no-no on the weight and fat loss program but, as occasional uses, these are permissible on the maintenance program.

You have reprogramed yourself off fried foods. You have reprogramed yourself off pizzas, pastas, pies, etc. You are programed to enjoy natural methods of cooking nourishing, high protein foods. Don't let yourself slip back to these old fattening ways.

Maintenance indicates that in order to maintain your peace of mind as a slender, attractive person, you must maintain your new eating program. It's now just a wee bit broader. If you made it more than a wee bit broader, you would be more than a wee bit broader yourself.

Scan these recipes now. I'll rejoin you in a few pages.

LUSTY SOUPS

Cucumber Vichyssoise (For 4)

2 C Buttermilk	1/3 C White Wine
2 Eggs, beaten	1 1/3 C Chopped Cucumber
2/3 T Chopped Celery Leaves	½ t Dried Dill Weed
1½ T Chopped Green Onions	Dash Freshly Ground Pepper
2/3 C Chicken Broth	Salt to taste

Heat milk gently, stirring in beaten eggs, green onion and celery until mixture coats a spoon. Stir in remaining ingredients and cook a few minutes longer. Chill and serve or blend in blender to a smooth creamy mixture, chill and serve.

Blender Gazpacho (For 3-4)

2-3 Sprigs Green Onions
1 Small Clove Garlic, peeled
2 Large Tomatoes, chopped
1 Small Green Pepper, seeded
1 Large Cucumber, sliced
½ t Oregano
Pinch of Thyme

1 T Salad Oil (optional)
1¼ T Cider Vinegar
1¼ T Lemon Juice
Salt and Pepper
½ C Chicken Broth
Parsley or Chinese Parsley
    as Garnish

Blend until smooth in blender. Chill and serve garnished with parsley.

Supper Soup (For 4)

4 C Strong Meat or
    Vegetable Stock
2/3 C Raw Spinach, chopped
2/3 C Chopped Onion
2/3 C Chopped Mixed Green
    Vegetables

1 Stalk Celery and
    Leaves, chopped
½ C Buttermilk
2 Eggs
Dash of Thyme

Gently boil stock and add greens and simmer, covered for about one hour. Gradually add buttermilk, stirring constantly until smooth. Add beaten eggs and continue cooking for another couple of minutes, stirring. Serve with a sprinkle of thyme in each bowl.

Hot Beef Soup (For 4)

1 lb. Lean Chopped Beef
½ C Chopped Celery
½ C Chopped Green Pepper,
    seeded
½ C Chopped Onion

1 Small Clove Garlic, minced
4 C Tomato Juice
Pinch of Oregano
½ C Chopped Green Vegetables,
    fresh or frozen

In Teflon pan, brown the meat. Add celery, green pepper, onion and garlic. Add tomato juice and vegetables. Simmer for about 40 minutes. Season with oregano, salt, and pepper to taste and serve.

SAVORY VEGETABLES

Onion Rings

3 Large Mild Onions, very
    thinly sliced
Dash Worcestershire Sauce

Water to cover
Chopped Watercress or
    Parsley to garnish

Bake in shallow pan, covered with water at 300 degrees until soft. Season and garnish.

Italian Green Beans (For 3-4)

1 pkg. Frozen Italian style
  Green Beans
1 Strip Bacon (lean)
1 Stalk Chopped Green
  Onion (top only)
1 Small Tomato, chopped

1 T Green Pepper, chopped
1 Small Clove Garlic, pressed
¼ t Oregano
Dash freshly Ground Black
  Pepper
Salt to season

Thaw beans partially. Saute bacon, adding green pepper, onion and garlic until lightly browned. Stir in all other ingredients. Add a little water and cover. Simmer until tender.

Asparagus Buca Lapi (For 2-3)

1 Frozen pkg. Asparagus
1½ T Water

Salt and Pepper to taste
Parmesan Cheese, grated

Cook quickly in covered pan. Watch to see that it does not overcook. Sprinkle with grated Parmesan cheese and season with salt and pepper.

Oven Baked Tomato with Green Spinach Sauce (For 2)

1 Large Tomato, halved
3/4 lb. Raw Spinach
2 T Chopped Green Onion

¼ C Skim Milk
Pinch of Basil Leaves
1 Sprig Parsley, chopped

Wash spinach and heat until wilted. Place in blender with a little milk and blend until smooth. Pour back into pan, add chopped green onion and simmer for about 3 minutes. Meanwhile, place tomato halves on pan and bake at 400 degrees until tender. Place spinach on top, sprinkle with basil and heat. Serve at once.

HEALTHFUL SALADS

Tomato and Bacon Salad (For 4)

Washed and Crisped
  Salad Greens
1 Mild Onion, cut in rings
½ C Low-calorie Dressing
¼ t Basil Leaves

5 Slices Crisp, Cooked
  Bacon, crumbled
2 Hard-boiled Eggs, sliced
2-3 Tomatoes, sliced

In separate bowls, arrange onion rings and tomato slices on greens. Stir basil into dressing and pour over salad. Sprinkle bacon on top and garnish with egg slices.

Cottage Cheese and Pineapple Salad (For 3)

2 oz. Cottage Cheese	1 T Wheat Germ
3 Slices Canned Sugar-free	Lettuce Leaves
Pineapple	Low-calorie Dressing
1 T Pineapple Juice	¼ C Bleu Cheese, crumbled

Combine cheese, juice and wheat germ. Shape into small balls. Place pineapple slices on lettuce top with cheese balls. Sprinkle with dressing and bleu cheese.

Luncheon Salad (For 6)

Small Head Lettuce, broken into bite-sized pieces	½ lb. Finely sliced Luncheon Meat, Ham or Chicken
1 Small Jar Hearts of Palms, Artichoke Hearts or Asparagus Tips	1 Hard-cooked Egg, cut into wedges
1 Stalk of Celery, finely sliced	¼ C Chopped Green Onions
	½ C Raw Cauliflower, finely sliced
	½ C Low-calorie Dressing

Rub inside of large wood bowl with garlic and discard. Combine all other ingredients. Toss lightly with dressing.

Low Calorie Salad Dressing

1 Clove Garlic, pressed	½ t Vinegar
Dash of Worcestershire Sauce	½ t Lime Juice
½ C Cottage Cheese	Dash of freshly ground
½ C Tomato Juice	Pepper

Place all ingredients in blender and whirl until smooth. Chill and use over all salads.

DELICIOUS ENTREES

Crabmeat Parisienne (For 4)

1 T Salad Oil	1¼ oz. Brandy
1 lb. Shredded Aged Cheddar type Cheese	1 lb. Crabmeat

Warm the oil and add cheese and brandy. Simmer until cheese is melted and smooth. Add crabmeat and stir gently until heated. Thin with skim milk if necessary and season with salt and freshly ground pepper. Serve on toasted whole wheat bread.

Meat and Cheese Loaf (For 5)

1 Onion, sliced
1 lb. Chopped Beef (low
    fat content)
1 C Tomato Juice
1 Bay Leaf, crushed
1 t Oregano Leaves

½ t Basil Leaves
1 Small Container Cottage
    Cheese
¼ lb. Jack or Cheddar
    Cheese, slivered
Salt and Pepper to taste

Brown meat and onion and pour off fat. Cover meat with tomato juice and seasonings and simmer for about 15 minutes. In loaf pan, layer meat, cottage cheese and slivered cheese. Repeat and top with cheese slivers. Cover with aluminum foil and bake at 400 degrees until cheese is melted. Remove foil and brown at 500 degrees for a couple of minutes.

West Coast Chicken Salad (For 4)

Dash of Chervil
1 t Poppy Seeds
¼ C Orange Juice
¼ C Low-calorie French
    dressing
1 3/4 C Cooked Cubed Chicken

2 Naval Oranges
1 Large Green Pepper,
    cut into rings
1 Small Mild Onion, sliced
Salad Greens
Pimento for Garnish

Mix together first 4 ingredients. Peel and slice oranges. Toss dressing lightly with chicken, oranges and onion. Chill for several hours. Arrange greens on platter. Top with green pepper rings and spoon on chicken mixture. Garnish with strips of pimento.

South China Shrimp and Beans

1½ lbs. Frozen raw, peeled,
    deveined Shrimp
1½ t Chicken Stock Base
1 C Boiling Water
¼ C Thinly Sliced Green
    Onion
1 Clove Garlic, crushed
1 T Salad Oil

1 t Salt
¼ t Ginger (powdered)
Dash Pepper
1 pkg. (9 ounces) Frozen
    Cut Green Beans
1 T Cornstarch
1 T Cold Water

Thaw frozen shrimp. Dissolve chicken stock base in boiling water. Cook onion, garlic, and shrimp in oil for 3 minutes, stirring frequently. If necessary, add a little of the chicken broth to prevent sticking. Stir in salt, ginger, pepper, green beans, and chicken broth. Cover and simmer 5 to 7 minutes longer or until beans are cooked but still slightly crisp. Combine cornstarch and water. Add cornstarch mixture to shrimp and cook until thick and clear, stirring constantly. Serves 6.

Fillets and Cabbage

1½ lbs. Fillets, fresh or frozen	2 T Sweet Pickle Relish
1 qt. Boiling Water	1 T Lemon Juice
1 T Salt	1 t Salt
¼ C Low Calorie Salad Dressing (mayonnaise type)	1 C Shredded Green Cabbage
	1 C Shredded Red Cabbage
	6 Lettuce Cups
2 T Chopped Onion	Lemon Wedges

Thaw frozen fillets. Place fillets in boiling salted water. Cover and simmer about 10 minutes or until fish flakes easily when tested with a fork. Drain. Remove skin and bones; flake. Combine salad dressing, onion, relish, lemon juice, salt, and fish. Chill at least 1 hour to blend flavors. Add cabbage and toss lightly. Serve in lettuce cups. Serve with lemon wedges. Serves 6.

Crab Victor

2 pkgs. (6 ounces each) King Crab Meat or other crab meat, fresh, frozen, or	2 Chicken Bouillon Cubes
	3 Cups Boiling Water
	1 Cup Low Calorie French Dressing
2 Cans (6½ or 7½ ounces each) Crab Meat	6 Large Lettuce Cups
2 Celery Hearts or Palm Hearts	Pepper

Thaw frozen crab meat. Drain crab meat. Remove any remaining shell or cartilage. Cut crab meat into 1 inch pieces. Wash and trim celery hearts so that they are about 5 inches long. Cut each heart into thirds lengthwise. Place celery in a 10-inch fry pan. Dissolve bouillon cubes in boiling water and pour over celery. Cover pan and simmer for 10 to 15 minutes or until tender. Let celery cool in bouillon. Drain. Place celery in a shallow baking dish. Pour French dressing over celery and chill for at least 2 hours. Remove celery from dressing. Drain. Place in lettuce cups. Sprinkle with pepper. Place approximately ¼ cup crab meat on celery. Serves 6.

French Pot Roast (For 6)

7 lbs. Bottom Round	2 T Catsup
2 t Salt	2 T Wine Vinegar
3 T Olive Oil	1 C Red Dry Wine
4 Garlic Cloves, pressed	1 C Water
1 Small Onion	4 Peppercorns
5 Cloves	1 oz. Bitter Chocolate
2 Bay Leaves	3-4 Sprigs of Watercress
2 t Cinnamon	

Heat oil in deep pan. Salt meat and brown slightly on all sides. Pour off excess fat. Stick onion with cloves and add with all other ingredients except the chocolate. Cover and simmer for 3 hours until tender. Remove meat to serving plate. Add chocolate to gravy, adjust seasonings and simmer until thickened. Pour over meat and serve, garnished with watercress.

Chicken À la Queen (For 4)

1 2/3 C Cooked Chicken, cubed	Stuffed Green Olives for
½ C Cucumber, cut into	garnish
strips	3/4 C Plain Yogurt
¼ C Celery, finely sliced	2 t Lime Juice
¼ C Radishes, sliced	Pinch of Marjoram
1 Medium Green Pepper, cut	1 Clove Garlic, squeezed
into rings	Salad Greens

Arrange pepper rings on greens. Combine all other ingredients and chill. Spoon onto pepper rings. Garnish with olives and more radishes.

Chicken Tarragon (For 4)

2 (2 lb.) Fryer Chickens,	1 t Dried Leaf Tarragon
halved	2 T Lime Juice
¼ t Worcestershire Sauce	1 t Catsup

Pull off skin and place chicken halves in shallow pan. Combine other ingredients and brush over both sides of chicken. Bake at 375 degrees for 3/4 of an hour, turning once.

DESSERTS

Almond Pudding (For 2)

2 T (2 envelopes) Knox
   gelatin
4 T Cold Water
1 C Boiling Water
1 t Vanilla

1 t Almond Extract
2/3 C Dry Non-fat Milk Powder
2 Envelopes Artificial Sugar
   Substitute
1½ C Crushed Ice

Sprinkle gelatin in cold water. Add to boiling water and stir until dissolved. In blender place gelatin mixture, dry milk, vanilla, almond and sugar. Blend for about 1 minute then add ice and blend until smooth. Chill and serve.

Raspberry Bavarian Creme (For 6)

1 pkg. Raspberry Low-calorie
   Dessert
1 C Boiling Water

1 C Cold Water (or 8
   ice cubes)
4 oz. Cottage Cheese

Add gelatin to boiling water and stir until completely dissolved. Add cold water or ice cubes and chill until thickened. Then add cottage cheese and beat or blend until smooth. Refrigerate until set.

Zabaglione (For 2)

4 Egg Yolks
4 T Dry Red Wine

2 Envelopes Artificial Sugar
   Substitute

Place ingredients over medium heat and bring to simmer while beating constantly until thick and fluffy. Serve in sherbet glasses, warm or chilled.

Raw Applesauce (For 1)

1 Cut-up Cored Apple
Liquid Sugar Substitute

1/3 C Unsweetened Apple
   Juice

Blend in blender all together and serve. Sprinkle with cinnamon.

YOUR PHYSICIAN'S ROLE ON YOUR
MAINTENANCE PROGRAM

Earlier in this chapter I cited the problems, the changes, and the crises of life as critical weight control times.

These are the times when emotional pressures can become great enough to force you out of newly created, healthful eating habits and back onto that old fattening escape to food, if you permit.

This is the time to think, identify, write and reprogram.

It may also be a good time to see your physician for a check-up.

Annual or semi-annual check-ups are a good procedure to follow. But during these times of pressure, it would be a wise move to throw in a precautionary visit.

When my patients leave—I often think of them as graduates—and embark on the maintenance program, I advise them to plan on at least three follow-up visits the first year.

I also prescribe additional medication when necessary only if there is a weight increase. These include hunger suppressants for hunger control and water tablets for reduction of excess body fluids. These are to be used only in the event of a sudden and excessive weight increase and then only until the base weight is restored.

Your own physician may want to see you are given similar aids on your weight maintenance program.

I hope more physicians will see obesity as a medical and emotional problem, one that requires both physiological and psychological attention. Fat is a symptom. The trouble could be that the body is malfunctioning, but more likely it is caused ultimately by emotional dysfunctioning. Doctors need to see past the scales into the patient's work, social life, and family. They should use simple applied psychology.

In this book I have strived to have you *do* for yourself. Now, I'm not lilly white on that score myself. I couldn't possibly help all my patients dig to the root of the matter. So I teach them how to do-it-yourself.

IT MUST TAKE NO MORE THAN THREE POUNDS
TO PUSH THE PANIC BUTTON

The scale and you will remain very close friends from now on. In fact, maintenance requires even closer surveillance by weighing than weight loss. I told you that on the weight and fat loss program it doesn't matter whether a pound off is registered today or tomorrow and daily weighing is not as important as daily thinking and programing.

However, on the maintenance program you are now concerned about a pound gained and it is most important for you to detect that pound gained as soon as it happens. If you don't, there may be two, three, four pounds gained before you can do something to stem the tide.

When you reach your perfect weight, say 115 pounds, weigh yourself daily but don't be concerned if you go to 116, just be careful. Be concerned at 117, and institute even greater care (size of portions, amount of bread or liquor, fruit, vegetables, salad oil, etc.).

At 118 pounds, three pounds over your best weight, push the panic button. This means you *must* return to the original weight and fat loss program. Decrease the intake of the fruits and vegetables you had added and eliminate the fringe benefits of the maintenance program.

Usually the emergency is soon over. Do not declare it over at 117 or even 116. Take your weight down to its original 115 pound level before going ahead once again onto the maintenance program.

Remember the anti-social horrors of obesity you are risking.

As a doctor you can bet your boots I detect mouth odors, underarm odors and quite an assortment of body odors. But here's one thing I have noticed: Body odor levels are reduced as weight is reduced.

There was one woman—I won't even give you her initials—I could detect when she came in the front door even though I was in a rear consulting room. She was mousy, very tense and teary. She lost weight from 167 to 135 in seven months and her body odor disappeared.

Now you can say she began to take more prophylactic pride in herself, but she wasn't like those who changed their hair styles or bought more stylish clothes. She was still mousy, but less flagrantly fragrant.

THE ONE PROGRAMING THAT ACTS AS PROFILE INSURANCE

I hope I don't sound like a broken record in extolling the improvements of men and women, boys and girls who lose weight by, in effect, becoming their own psychologist. Take P.N., 17, 157 pounds and 5'6". Color her sloppy, nervous, loudspoken, obtrusive, slovenly and lazy.

The scene changes. It is eight weeks later. P.N. weighs 137. She is no longer nervous. She is confident and speaks with a well-modulated voice. She is coping like an adult with the usual pressures from home, school and friends. She's working part time, enjoys selling dresses, and is always tastefully dressed herself. Best of all, P.N. makes decisions and carries them out. She reached her weight goal and she will reach her goals in life.

"Eating properly activates my mind. I do my work smarter. Sex is better as I feel calmer and more desirable. I'm less bloated when I eat and have less problems with gas. My skin is more youthful. I'm now a happy, contented woman." I hear it again and again.

As I write, I see a report in front of me from K.I., a housewife with three children. She is writing about herself after eight weeks on the program.

"My weight so far is 21 pounds less with a total of 10½ inches gone from my bust, waist, hips and thighs.
"I have had a condition in the knees a doctor told me could turn into arthritis. Since I have been eating properly, I have no pain in my knees. This is miraculous."

Read this report and see if you can guess the age bracket of the woman who wrote it:

"I began the weight control program in April of 1973 and weighed 159 pounds. Five months later I now weigh 120 pounds and feel like a human instead of an overstuffed pig.
"Here are some physical changes I've noticed:
1. Blood pressure normal.
2. Varicose veins are disappearing and there is no more pain.
3. I can now play tennis, ride a bicycle and walk more without my legs and muscles aching.
4. My skin has cleared.
5. I have no shortness of breath. I do not become tired, weak or fatigued. Headaches and backaches have disappeared.
6. My weight loss is 39 pounds. I feel and look great. I've lost 3 inches in the bust, 4 inches in the waist, and 6 inches in the hips. I am now wearing a size 12 dress, down from a size 16.
"My emotional benefits are immense. I can mix with others and have just as much fun without becoming too nervous and irritable. I don't have the fear, guilt or shame that I had before going on the weight control program.
"My husband was drifting away from me. I didn't care as I had an inferiority complex about myself, such as being heavy and out of shape,

no pep to go where he suggested (I was too tired to get dressed.) and sex was a dirty word to me. But, mention food and I was never too tired to eat. After being on this weight control program, my how I have changed. It's just like being on my first honeymoon!"

This patient achieved many physical and emotional changes through relaxation and imagining (visualizing). These ingredients are essential steps in this miracle weight loss guide. This woman was 61 when she wrote this. Nonetheless, losing almost 40 pounds certainly permitted her to enjoy life all over again.

You have acquired a very valuable skill on the weight and fat loss program. You have learned to program yourself.

To do this, you quieted the body and the mind—very deeply. Then you held certain images in your mind's eye.

These visual thoughts become things. You can use this programing to accomplish *any* goal you desire to attain in the years ahead—including the goal of maintaining your attractiveness and perfect weight, on and on.

Keep in practice. Program yourself daily for this perfect weight and youthful look.

HOW TO: KEEP IN TRIM WITH A MENTAL IMAGE

1. Relax your body and quiet your mind at bed time.
2. Review your eating for the day, giving yourself a mental pat on the back for aspects well done.
3. Hold in your mind's eye the picture of yourself slender as you are now—energetic, youthful, popular, successful.
4. End your session on the count of 1-2-3.

If, before you end each session on the count of three, you say to yourself, "Next time I will go deeper, faster," soon you will no longer have to go through any procedure to reach that tranquil state. The moment you sit in that straight backed chair you are *there*, ready for productive imagining (visualizing).

I know some who have become so expert at this they can take a moment off at their office desk, even in an elevator, to reinforce their programing for energy, creativity, influence, desire for fresh, clean air in their lungs (anti-smoking), and desire for high protein, high nutrition foods in their belly (anti-blubber).

THE "BIG" PERSON YOU REALLY ARE

All over the country today, people are taking great interest in a whole new family of activities. Here are just a few of them:

Hatha Yoga, Bio-Feedback Training, Executive Power Seminars, Encounter Groups, Zen, T-Groups, Sensitivity Training, Human Potential Groups, Meditation, Psychocybernetics, Psychosynthesis, Body Dynamics, Achievement Motivation, Creative Conflict, etc.

Basically, what they are all doing is learning to know themselves better. Obviously, there is no one way to do this.

One fact is absolutely certain: The better you know and understand yourself, the better able you are to acquire whatever you seek out of life, to give whatever you desire, and to become the person you want to be.

I have given you a way to know yourself. You don't have to join a group. You work alone with *you*.

The way I have given you has been proven successful.

Hundreds of formerly stout men are now free of their abdominal protrusion and stand lithe and erect.

Hundreds of formerly roly-poly women are now experiencing the admiration of men.

Hundreds of pairs of flapping thighs, bouncing jowls, bobbing buttocks, and billowing bosoms are now normalized. Double and triple chins are now unified, slumping stomachs are flattened, and miscellaneous bulges beautified.

There are thousands of sets of before and after pictures to demonstrate this. I don't keep them. I return them to my patients because it is more important that they have them, to keep, to remind and to motivate.

The way I have given you to know yourself *works*. It works off your unwanted fat permanently. It is a way of thought, not diet.

There is only one kind of fat that it won't touch: Fat between the ears. A fat-headed person who refuses to think about himself, to learn to know himself, to love himself, is doomed to diet discipline.

On the other hand, think and you shrink without a moment of growling stomach or hunger pangs.

Have a steak.

Have a chicken leg.
Have a hard-boiled egg.
But, above all, *have a thought.*

One day, this easy method of weight control may be taught in medical schools. Believe me, I would jump with joy if that day arrives. They don't even have to call it the Doctor Schiff Method.

I would be delighted, too, when the day arrives, and arrive it must, when they teach thought and understanding about self to high-school students and university students, including the helpful techniques of writing and reprograming for goal reaching and success.

But above all, I would be thrilled if this book has taught you how to reach your weight goal and stay slim by knowing yourself. I would be doubly thrilled if this book has helped you to understand your emotional "being" and to achieve your miracle.

I have come to feel very close to you, writing *to* you this way. I hope you will not lend me to someone else, but will keep me near you so you will always have the "HOW TO" for being slim, so you will always be able to open these pages and be encouraged to think about yourself as a way of life.

It is a beautiful life. When you awaken each morning, think how beautiful it actually is.

Think about how beautiful and wonderful you really are.

Think about those who love you.

And love yourself.